MIDWIFERY

EXCELLENCE IN NURSING
THE RESEARCH ROUTE

MIDWIFERY

Edited by

ANN FAULKNER

PhD, MLitt, MA, SRN, RCNT, DipEd
Professor of Communication in Health Studies, Sheffield University, and
Deputy Director, Trent Regional Palliative and Continuing Care Centre

and

TRICIA MURPHY-BLACK

PhD, MSc, RGN, RM, RCNT
Research Fellow, University of Edinburgh

SCUTARI PRESS
London

First published 1990

British Library Cataloguing in Publication Data:
Midwifery
    1. Great Britain. Midwifery
    I. Faulkner, Ann II. Murphy – Black, Tricia III.
    Series 610.73678

ISBN 1-871364-31-0

Typeset by Inforum Typesetting, Portsmouth
Printed and bound in Great Britain by
The Alden Press, Oxford, London and Northampton

CONTENTS

CONTRIBUTORS

Ros Bryar, BNurs, MPhil, SRN, HV, NDN, SCM
Lecturer in Continuing Education, University College of Swansea, and West Glamorgan Health Authority

Jean Davies, SRN, SCM, MSc
Community Midwife, Princess Mary Maternity Hospital, Newcastle-upon-Tyne

Frances Evans, BA, PhD
Senior Policy Research Officer, Newcastle City Council

Ann Faulkner, PhD, MLitt, MA, SRN, RCNT, DipEd
Professor of Communication in Health Studies, Sheffield University and Deputy Director, Trent Regional Palliative and Continuing Care Centre

Jenifer Holden, MPhil(Edin), BSc(Hons), SRN, HV
Research Associate, Department of Nursing Studies, University of Edinburgh, and Psychology Lecturer, Queen Margaret College, Edinburgh

Penny Jones, SRN, SCM, ADM
Midwifery Sister, Countess of Chester Hospital, Chester

Glynis Mayes, BSc, SRN, SCM, NDN, HV Dip
Maternity and Paediatric Services, Whipps Cross Hospital, Waltham Forest Health Authority

Tricia Murphy Black, PhD, MSc, RGN, RM, RCNT
Research Fellow, University of Edinburgh

Kate Niven, PhD, BSc, RGN
Lecturer in Psychology, Glasgow College of Technology

Jennifer Sleep, SRN, SCM, MTD, BA
District Research Coordinator, West Berkshire Health Authority

Peter Wright, MA, DPhil, CPsychol, FBPS
Lecturer in Psychology, University of Edinburgh

PREFACE

Research in nursing is now well established, very much in line, in one respect, with the recommendations of the Briggs Report (Briggs, 1979) that nursing as a research-based profession should have some nurses who specialise in research. The second criterion, that all nurses should be research minded, has yet to occur. There are many reasons for this.

First, a belief has arisen that researchers in nursing see themselves as an elite group. Journals such as the *Nursing Times* have described researchers as academics in ivory towers, and it is not uncommon for the correspondence columns of journals to carry criticism of researchers, suggesting that they are unaware of the real world.

Second, there is hostility to those who, by the very nature of their research, appear to be criticising current practice. It is not uncommon, when describing uncomfortable results, to be told, 'It couldn't happen where *I* work.' This, even when more than one study suggests the same pattern of results.

Third, research in nursing is often called into question because change does not necessarily occur as a result. This may be because there is not yet enough evidence for change, or because the research was descriptive and therefore did not offer solutions, or indeed because change happens slowly no matter how overwhelming the evidence. It may also be that research results are not disseminated to the profession.

'Excellence in Nursing: the research route' was conceived in the belief that the majority of nurses are committed to improving patient care and that research findings can be an aid in that improvement – not only by offering solutions but also by critically questioning practice. This questioning may be described as 'research-mindedness' and, hopefully, can be developed in all nurses.

A further belief is that there *is* a gulf between those who research and those who practise. The ivory tower myth needs to be dispelled. One of the problems may lie in the traditional language of research, which has a jargon of its own. That clinical nurses do not understand this language is no more surprising than that a researcher unfamiliar with critical care should not understand the language of an intensive care unit.

Another problem may well lie in the natural defensiveness of health professionals who believe that they are being criticised by researchers. It is unfortunate that, so often, findings that show clear deficits of care should be taken personally, when the real problem may be within the system itself. Communication is a case in point, where study after study confirms problems in nurse–patient relationships. However, these appear to be linked less with nurses' unwillingness to communicate than with a deficit in teaching professional communication skills. Once research can be seen in terms of its relevance *to the profession* rather than its inherent criticism of individual practice, hopefully there will be less hostility to those who research.

This series aims to present research in a way that makes sense to clinical nurses. That is not to say that it is oversimplified – rather that the papers are clearly presented and interesting to read. This volume on midwifery explores some areas that, hopefully, will be of interest to those 'at the sharp end' – maybe because they spark ideas or perhaps give a feeling of *déjà vu*. The writers range from clinical nurses who have taken time out for research to those whose major involvement is in research.

To assess the relevance of research to reality, the final chapters are written by a clinical practitioner and a manager, for it is not researchers who will bring change, but those who practise and are research minded.

I am particularly pleased to have Tricia Murphy-Black as co-editor of this volume. She has made her own contribution to excellence in midwifery, and I have always found her a pleasure to work with.

Ann Faulkner

REFERENCE

Briggs, A. (1979) *Royal Commission on the National Health Service*. London: HMSO.

1

INTRODUCTION

Tricia Murphy-Black and Ann Faulkner

Care of the childbearing woman has been subject to considerable change over the past 50 years. The members of the multidisciplinary team who care for mothers and babies would agree that the aim of these changes is to reduce the risk of death and morbidity. The means of providing this care, however, has been the subject of debate, dispute and widely differing views. Midwives and obstetricians – the two professions most closely concerned with caring for the pregnant woman and her child – have changed their practices many times in that half century. What was considered to be a high standard of care yesterday is questioned today and by tomorrow may be regarded not merely as old-fashioned but also as dangerous. These changes have come about by increasing knowledge, which has been derived from a variety of sources, such as medical research, technological advances, consumer demands and, in the past few years, midwives' research.

Obstetricians, although numerically the smaller of the two professions, have the power to influence treatment and to decide what it should be, where it should be carried out, by whom and how. Although of a high standard and organised, and with a tradition of research, their knowledge, like all knowledge, has grown step by step. The management or treatment that has resulted from this knowledge has sometimes been revealed later as being less of a benefit than was first supposed.

One example of a treatment, widely used in both the UK and the USA in the 1940s, was the administration of diethylstilboestrol (DES) to prevent spontaneous abortion. The critical evaluation of this drug did not take long enough, and it was only with the next generation that the consequence of a significant increase in the incidence of carcinoma of the vagina was appreciated (Apfel and Fisher, 1986). The other drug with well-known effects when given to pregnant women – thalidomide – is still considered safe in the non-pregnant.

Technological advances that have changed the patterns of care of the mother in labour have included electronic foetal monitoring (EFM). Machines for foetal monitoring, developed in the 1960s, started to be part of standard labour ward equipment in the 1970s. By the end of the 1970s, the use of monitors was seen not only as a means of reducing perinatal mortality but also as part of the armament to safeguard against legal action if the parents should decide to sue. Not all agreed, however, with the widespread use of EFM. Inch (1982), in an adaptation of MacLennan's 'cascade of intervention', includes EFM within the model that contributes to the morbidity of mother and baby. In a large, randomised controlled trial of EFM and intermittent auscultation with nearly 13 000 mothers, Macdonald et al

(1985) reported no differences between the two groups in stillbirth and neonatal death rates, congenital abnormalities, the incidence of low Apgar scores at 5 minutes of age and neonatal infections. Although some of the findings were conflicting, the authors' subsequent policy is to restrict the use of EFM to those mothers who have specific indications of risk.

Changes in obstetric practice influenced by consumer groups include the induction of labour. The increase in the incidence of induction in the early 1970s was such that the reasons for it were challenged by some consumer groups, and consequently the media were suspicious that it was more for the benefit of hospital staff than of mother or baby. A drop in the rate of surgical induction at one London hospital from 31.4% in 1971 to 19.3% in 1975 (Prince and Adams, 1978) may have been coincidence or may have been influenced by the television and newspaper attention to this issue in 1974. Such an impact of consumer groups could only come about because they were well organised. This organisation is a feature of post-war Britain with both the National Childbirth Trust (NCT) and the Association for the Improvement of Maternity Services (AIMS), as well as others, starting in a small way and growing in the past 40 years.

Research into the clinical practice of midwives by midwives is a recent phenomenon. Despite their claim through the years that midwives are practitioners in their own right, many of their practices have developed with little or no research. While obstetricians may have embarked on some treatments that were later demonstrated to be inadequately evaluated or tested, midwives have scant documented evidence for some aspects of their care. Until recently some textbooks have repeated the same traditions without any references (Myles, 1975, 1985). The care given by midwives could be put into three categories:

1. practices that are part of the received wisdom handed on from one generation of midwives to the next;
2. fashionable dogma that follows a trend without questioning;
3. medical prescription.

The impact of these on midwifery practice can be illustrated by the following examples.

During the 1970s, when the incidence of breast feeding was low, midwives were taught to control how mothers breast fed their babies. To prevent cracked nipples, Myles (1975, p. 458) states that 'midwives should not allow' babies to suck for longer than 3 minutes on each breast every 6 hours of the first 24 hours of life. As this statement is unreferenced it is difficult to know the basis for the practice, especially as the physiology of lactation was well-established and readily available in the paperback edition of Gunther's book *Infant Feeding* (1973, first published 1971). It is possible that it was derived from a misinterpretation of Gunther's earlier (1945) research. She demonstrated the increased negative pressure when a baby was at the breast but not sucking: 'Greater negative pressures were recorded in other instances, and one two-day-old baby exerted a suction of 200mmHg for 2 min. until she was removed from the breast. The outward appearance of the baby gave no indication of the strength of negative pressure obtaining; indeed the contrast was striking between the peaceful child apparently at rest on the breast and the high level of negative pressure recorded by the instrument'. Gunther's summary was that a petechial lesion was mainly caused by suction unrelieved by swallowing. As a result she recommended: 'To prevent the petechial type [lesion] the child should not be left on the breast for more than 2 min. *when it is obtaining nothing*' (emphasis added). It may be questioned whether or not the practice of restricting the length of time at the breast grew from the first part of the last quote, without an appreciation of the significance of the last five words. If this is so, many mothers may have had an unnecessary struggle to establish breast feeding.

Although Romney (1982) would classify pre-delivery shaving as a traditional practice, her review of its history demonstrates the interaction between the publicity given by Mr Gillette to his safety razor and the short skirts and silk stockings worn in the 1920s, which could classify this practice as fashionable dogma. Romney questions whether or not perineal shaving would have been accepted by mothers if the only means of doing it was using the cut-throat razor. Once the routine was established, the research evidence of a lower incidence of puerperal fever in unprepared mothers (Johnson and Siddall, 1922) was ignored. For 60 years, only those who arrived in hospital late in labour escaped the pre-delivery shave. It is encouraging that midwives, despite their tradition of unquestioning acceptance, can change their practice. A recent preliminary report (Garcia et al, 1986) of a 1984 survey involving 193 English health districts noted that only 1% of consultant units carried out a complete shave, while an additional 37% did a partial shave.

Midwifery practice that is controlled by medical prescription includes the artificial rupture of the amniotic membranes. Henderson (1984) demonstrated in a small study that the midwives who performed this procedure deceived themselves about the reasons for rupturing membranes. They reported they had more autonomy in the decision-making than they actually had. Their decisions were, in fact, either directly or indirectly influenced by the medical staff. In addition, the midwives who were observed ruptured the membranes without consulting the mother.

The above examples show that some midwifery practice is derived from received wisdom, fashion and medical prescription. There must be many mothers who have suffered at the hands of midwives – those with sore nipples for whom breast feeding became a painful battleground or was reluctantly abandoned; those who suffered discomfort from unnecessary pubic shaving; and those who had the amniotic membranes ruptured without their consent. This may seem minimal suffering when contrasted with the effect of DES in causing vaginal carcinoma. It can be questioned, however, which profession is the more culpable. Obstetricians who gave DES did so in the belief that it would save the pregnancy – all the knowledge that was available at the time. Midwives were in a different position; they restricted feeding times and removed pubic hair despite evidence that these interventions were harmful. Both of these interventions were taught to midwives, who accepted and carried them out. As a product of training in the 1970s the author herself was a 'good' midwife and dutifully did both, using as much charm and authority as she could to persuade mothers that these were 'right'.

If midwives want to claim their status as independent practitioners or wish to be held accountable for their own practice, they should know not only what they must do and how to do it but also why they do it. It is only by constantly questioning what is done and how it is done that midwives can build up a body of knowledge on which to base their practice. This knowledge will grow step by step; what is accepted today as 'good' practice may have to be discarded tomorrow when increasing knowledge shows the flaws.

As more and more mothers are themselves questioning what a midwife does, it is essential that a midwife can support her actions with research evidence. The mother who refuses to have an injection of Syntometrine after delivery of the baby may be basing her decision on books aimed at encouraging women to be more active in their health care. Statements such as 'suckling the baby after the birth can effectively expel the placenta but this is rarely allowed . . . Herbal remedies such as angelica can help with the expulsion of the placenta and thus obviate the need for injections' (Phillips and Rakusen, 1978) encourage mothers to make such a demand. This puts the midwife in an invidious position. On the one hand, she is expected to carry out the doctor's standing orders (to give Syntometrine routinely) yet, on the other, the mother refuses to be given it. Although (or perhaps because) midwives do carry out procedures without a mother's express permission, in this instance they are forestalled in advance. Nowhere in this situation can the midwife exercise her own clinical judgment. Does she have any evidence of the benefits of this intervention? Does she have any evidence of hazard if she does not do it? Knowledge of this sort presented to a mother may help to resolve the situation, with the mother agreeing to the exercise of clinical judgment. This is a different situation from a confrontation where one side refuses and all the other side can say is that she had been told to give it.

If the midwifery profession had always been research-based with all practices questioned and the evidence documented through the years, and if midwives were always able to give the pros and cons of what they were doing, maybe the profession would not have to be so concerned today about loss of status as an independent practitioner. It is certainly too late and perhaps unfair to expect that there should be such a tradition of midwifery research. The roots of this lack lie in the poor opportunities for education and the position of women as well as midwives in society. The struggle to secure legislation of midwives in the late nineteenth and early twentieth centuries 'to reduce unnecessary suffering and loss of life . . . also to ensure for the midwife a high level of competence and respect appropriate to her calling' (Withams, 1985) was as much as could be expected at that time.

It may be too late to *have* a tradition of midwifery research but it is not too late to *start* one. If all midwifery practice is required to have a research base, it needs considerable commitment from the profession. All midwives need to be research minded. This has implications for the future development of clinical midwives, midwife teachers and midwife managers. This commitment will require that the research-minded midwife at the bedside will not only base her practice on research findings but also have the skills to evaluate critically the research of others. She will be able to judge whether a particular research report is worth following up or whether the limitations of the study are such that the results cannot be generalised. Even if it seems that the results can be generalised, carrying out replication studies will add to the body of knowledge as well as answering specific questions about a particular group of mothers or a local practice. The findings may be supported or challenged; either way it will help to make decisions about implementation.

Midwife teachers will not only use research findings as the basis for their everyday teaching but will also encourage their students to learn about the research process. Part of this learning could be the carrying out of a project. In order to do this, the teachers themselves need to have a good working knowledge of research methods so that they can guide their students (Royal College of Midwives, 1987). While the teachers may well draw on the educational research of other disciplines, they will also have a role in carrying out research in midwifery education. This will be necessary if good use is to be made of the opportunities to experiment with different forms of training (NT Newsfocus, 1987).

The research interests of midwife managers will be different but complementary. One vital role is to aid the clinical midwife in her evaluation of research reports. In order to do this managers need both experience of clinical practice and knowledge of research. If change in practice is to follow evaluation of research findings, considerable management skills are required to allow this change to take place. As a member of a multidisciplinary team, a midwife's actions impinge on those of others. Before a change in practice can be accepted the managers will have to negotiate, not only with their own staff but also with the other members of the team. They also have a responsibility to help to facilitate research. This may take the form of arrangements that allow members of their staff time and facilities to carry out research projects. It may also involve employing others to carry out research projects. Part of this skill may include writing proposals and seeking funding.

There is another responsibility of midwife managers that is theirs alone: acting as a gateway to research. There are few projects that do not require their permission and their power should be used wisely. Managers who refuse to allow research to be undertaken in their unit may be frustrating an individual, but for the research base of the profession as a whole and for the welfare of mothers and babies such refusal may have more serious implications. Conversely, the same managers have a duty to the mothers and babies in their unit to make sure they are not 'over-researched'. This may mean that they have to refuse access to the researchers. Sometimes both needs can be accommodated by ensuring that projects take place at different times so that no one group of mothers is inconvenienced by a surfeit of researchers.

The research in this book covers only a few of the many skills that midwives and others need. Indeed, it is only a part of the relevant research, and there is still much to be done. Research into midwives' practice and the practice of other members of the multidisciplinary team is a start towards building up the knowledge needed to reassure mothers that we are giving the best possible care. As with DES, induction of labour, foetal monitoring, breast feeding and pubic shaving, the findings presented here may be demonstrated in later years as inaccurate or only part of the truth. If they are only part of the truth, the rest of it will only be discovered if this book is read with critical attention. If every statement is questioned and challenged, if the flaws in the projects are discovered (for few projects are perfect), then the midwifery profession is starting to grow up. If, however, this questioning, this challenging, leads to a total disregard of all the findings and to an inability to see the values despite the limitations, the growth will be stunted, and eventually it is mothers and babies who will suffer. On the other hand, if the research available now is used as a foundation to build on, so that the knowledge becomes a high mountain, future midwives will be able to stand on the top and see much further than we can today. They may feel superior with their increased knowledge in comparison with our limited vision, but they will not have a mountain to stand on if we do not start building it today.

REFERENCES

Apfel, R.J. and Fisher, S.M. (1986) *To Do No Harm: DES and the Dilemmas of Modern Medicine.* Yale: Yale University Press.

Garcia, J., Garforth, S. and Ayres, S. (1986) *The Policy and Practice in Midwifery Study: Progress Report.* MIDIRS Information Pack no. 2.

Gunther, M. (1945) Sore nipples: causes and prevention. *The Lancet,* **ii**: 590–593.

Gunther, M. (1973) *Infant Feeding,* 2nd edn. Harmondsworth: Penguin.

Henderson, C. (1984) Influences and interactions surrounding the midwife's decision to rupture the membranes. *Research and the Midwife Conference Proceedings,* pp. 68–85. London: King's College.

Inch, S. (1982) *Birthrights: A Parents' Guide to Modern Childbirth.* London: Hutchinson.

Johnson, R.A. and Siddall, R.S. (1922) Is the usual method of preparing patients for delivery beneficial or necessary? *American Journal of Obstetrics and Gynecology,* **4**: 645–650.

Macdonald, D., Grant, A., Sheridan Pereira, M., Boylan, P. and Chalmers, I. (1985) The Dublin randomised controlled trial of intra partum fetal heart rate monitoring. *American Journal of Obstetrics and Gynecology,* **152**(5): 524–539.

Myles, M. (1975) *Textbook for Midwives,* 8th edn. Edinburgh: Churchill Livingstone.

Myles, M. (1985) *Textbook for Midwives,* 10th edn. Edinburgh: Churchill Livingstone.

NT Newsfocus (1987) Ready for lift-off. *Nursing Times,* **83**(4): 16.

Phillips, A. and Rakusen, J. (1978) *Our Bodies, Our Selves: A Health Book by and for Women.* Harmondsworth: Penguin.

Prince, J. and Adams, M.E. (1978) *Minds, Mothers and Midwives: The Psychology of Childbirth.* Edinburgh: Churchill Livingstone.

Romney, M.L. (1982) Nursing research in obstetrics and gynaecology. *International Journal of Nursing Studies,* **19**: 193–203.

Royal College of Midwives (1987) *The Role and Education of the Future Midwife in the United Kingdom.* London: RCM.

Withams, S.C. (1985) *The Image of Midwives in the Nineteenth Century.* Unpublished dissertation, Sheffield City Polytechnic.

2

EPISIOTOMY

Jennifer Sleep

BACKGROUND TO THE STUDY

In recent years, midwives have become increasingly aware of the need to evaluate aspects of their care. This is especially true when considering the justification for intervention in the management of normal labour (Chalmers, 1989). The issues are emotive and often controversial, none more so than the subject of episiotomy and its role in the conduct of normal deliveries.

This controversy is fuelled by the concern of both practitioners and women and hinges on the conflicting rationale for practice as well as on the rapid rise in the frequency with which the procedure is being performed. Figures from maternity units in England and Wales demonstrate that the episiotomy rate for all deliveries doubled from 25% in 1967 to 53% in 1978 (Macfarlane and Mugford, 1984). It has been reported that this procedure is carried out on between 50 and 90% of women giving birth to their first child (Thacker and Banta, 1983).

The protagonists claim that the liberal use of the operation will reduce both serious vaginal and perineal tears as well as longer-term problems such as stress incontinence and vaginal prolapse (Donald, 1979; Flood, 1982). The antagonists claim that spontaneous trauma causes fewer problems than do the episiotomies that are done to prevent them (House, 1981; Kitzinger and Walters, 1981). These divergent views are reflected in a wide variation in rate of use of the operation, especially for maternal indications; there is less controversy relating to its use to alleviate foetal problems. This variance has been demonstrated on both an individual and a national basis; for example, the use of episiotomy by midwives working in one maternity unit was found to vary 10-fold (Wilkerson, 1984). In a national study conducted in 184 English maternity units in 1985, the episiotomy rate varied from 20 to 79% (Garcia et al, 1985). This highlights the disparity that occurs when clinical practice is based solely on clinical impression without the benefit of formal evaluation. As Chalmers (1984) emphasises, 'the costs of not assessing the validity of informal impressions about the effects of care using more formal evaluations can be high, both because effective forms of care are not recognised as promptly as possible, and also because forms of care that are ineffective or positively harmful are not detected efficiently.' The use of episiotomy represents such an issue.

Most midwives would claim that their decision of whether or not to perform an episiotomy is based on clinical judgment, but this is likely to include a fair measure of intuition, wish fulfilment and blind prejudice as well as personal experience and objective appraisal. What has been lacking is the scientific evidence on which practice can be based. A substantial review and analysis of over 350 books and articles published since 1870 in the English language literature on the subject concluded: 'There is no clearly defined evidence for its efficacy, particularly for routine use' (Thacker and Banta, 1983).

Several descriptive studies have assessed mothers' attitudes and experiences of pain following perineal trauma (Kitzinger and Walters, 1981; Cater, 1984). Groups of women managed by episiotomy have been compared with groups of women with perineal tears. One of the limitations of such design is that it is never possible to be sure that the groups being compared are similar in other important respects. It is obviously inappropriate to compare a large episiotomy performed to allow instrumental delivery with a vaginal tear sustained during a spontaneous birth. Furthermore, even if the comparison is restricted to normal vaginal deliveries, it should be recognised that those who have episiotomies are not necessarily comparable to those who sustain tears (the episiotomy may have been performed because it was judged that an extensive tear was imminent). Clearly, the most appropriate comparison is between groups of women similar in these and other respects but who sustain different patterns of trauma. Such comparability is best secured by using an 'experimental' or randomised controlled trial study design. By basing the allocation on a random selection, two groups are generated that are similar in respect both of factors, such as mode of delivery, known to be important and of factors unrecognised as potentially biasing, such as predisposition to extensive trauma.

Such an experimental study was designed to compare the liberal use of episiotomy with its restricted use in otherwise normal deliveries. The following hypotheses were tested, i.e. that the liberal use of episiotomy in normal deliveries reduces:

1. the incidence of severe tears at delivery;
2. the number of babies with low Apgar scores;
3. perineal pain in the puerperium;
4. the number of mothers reporting perineal pain 3 months following delivery;
5. the time to resumption of sexual intercourse;
6. the incidence of dyspareunia 3 months postpartum.

Ethical Considerations

In any experimental design there are important ethical considerations in dealing with human subjects. The conduct of a randomised controlled trial makes the intellectually honest admission that the best approach is not known and that the most ethical course of action is to find out which of the treatments under test is the better. At the same time, the risk of withholding the better treatment from the majority of patients is minimised.

A prerequisite is that informed consent is obtained. Because there is no consensus about what constitutes informed consent, this can be a difficult issue and one not easily resolved. What is paradoxical is that ethical questions seldom arise when new treatments, e.g. ultrasound as a diagnostic tool or as therapy, are introduced without any prior evaluation, yet once trials are designed to evaluate practice, protest on ethical grounds frequently ensues.

It was not considered acceptable that women's consent to participate in the study be invited on admission in labour; there is a great deal of stress and insufficient opportunity for discussion at this time. An informative letter was, therefore, distributed to all women when seen by the midwife either at the antenatal clinic or at home during the last trimester of pregnancy. Discussion was freely available and a contact telephone number given. Consent to participation was, therefore, implied unless stated to the contrary. In the event, only seven women refused to participate, requesting specific management. Their wishes for their own care were respected.

The protocol for the study discussed in this chapter was approved by the Research and Ethics committee for the West Berkshire Health District.

METHOD

The purpose of a randomised controlled trial is to allow unbiased comparison of methods of treatment (Chalmers, 1984). This demands meticulous attention to detail and scrupulous honesty at each stage of the design. There are a few golden rules (Grant, 1982):

1. *The allocation must not be predictable in advance.* If the investigator knows the treatment in advance, he or she may be tempted to arrange the order of entry to the study so that particular women receive one treatment rather than the other; this may be the one that the investigator considers to be the best, or he or she may choose to exclude a woman if the allocation is considered 'unsuitable'. Randomisation after entry is a way of minimising this risk. In this trial, entry was signalled by opening an opaque, sealed envelope. This was delayed until the midwife was confident of a normal, vaginal delivery; that is when delivery was imminent and she decided to scrub up. This also minimised the likelihood that a mother would need assistance by forceps or ventouse extraction, so making her ineligible for inclusion.

Each envelope contained a directive for one of two policies for managing the perineum, both aimed to minimise trauma:

a. *the restrictive policy* – the intention being that episiotomy should be restricted to foetal indications only;

b. *the liberal policy* – the intention being that the operation should be used more liberally to prevent a tear.

Thus there was never an absolute directive that an elective episiotomy should be performed on any mother; on the contrary, whatever the allocation, the midwife was asked to conduct the delivery without any trauma if at all possible.

Women were recruited concurrently to the two trial groups to ensure that conditions were as similar as possible for each of them; for example, they would be cared for by the same staff, on the same wards and by the same community midwives. Thus, it was hoped that, in most respects, each mother would receive similar midwifery care throughout the duration of the study.

2. *Each subject must have an equal chance of allocation to either of the treatments.* This eliminates selection bias at entry and ensures that the groups to be compared are similar at the onset of the study, any differences solely reflecting chance. Thus the numbered, sealed, envelopes containing the random allocation were allotted in sequence of admission. Women were eligible for entry if:

    a. they had a singleton foetus of at least 37 weeks gestational age, in a cephalic presentation;

    b. a spontaneous vaginal delivery was anticipated towards the end of the second stage of labour.

3. *There is no withdrawal of subjects once entered.* This controls for selection bias, which so often occurs in clinical trials. The groups, as randomised, differ only by chance; any subsequent withdrawals are likely to introduce bias because it is very unlikely that similar women will be withdrawn from each group. Thus once the envelope was opened, the mother had entered the trial regardless of subsequent management. If, however, the midwife failed to fulfil the trial directive, she was asked to note the reason; for the purpose of analysis the woman remained in the group to which she had been *allocated* because it is the randomised groups that are directly comparable.

A mediolateral incision was used throughout, in accordance with unit policy.

SAMPLE SIZE

The trial size was preset at 1000 women. Power calculations indicated that a trial of this size would have a 90% chance of finding a significant difference if, in truth, the restrictive policy doubled the incidence of an outcome expected in 5% of cases and a 95% power of detecting an increase of 50% in an outcome expected in 20% of cases.

The study was conducted in the West Berkshire Health District. For ease of supervision recruitment was restricted to consultant unit admissions only. During the 5-month study period in 1982, 1077 women met the entry criteria. Of these 77 were not recruited, either because delivery was precipitous or (sometimes) because the trial was forgotten. One thousand women, i.e. 93% of eligible mothers, were successfully recruited, and the study population may be considered representative of all vaginal deliveries in the hospital. During the study period there were 201 assisted deliveries and 62 caesarean sections of cephalic presentation, singleton babies of at least 37 weeks gestational age.

The student's t and chi squared tests were used to compare variables in the two groups. The design of the study is summarised in Figure 2.1.

DATA COLLECTION

The midwives were asked to note the time at which each envelope was opened. Descriptive data were collected on entry to the study. This included details such as

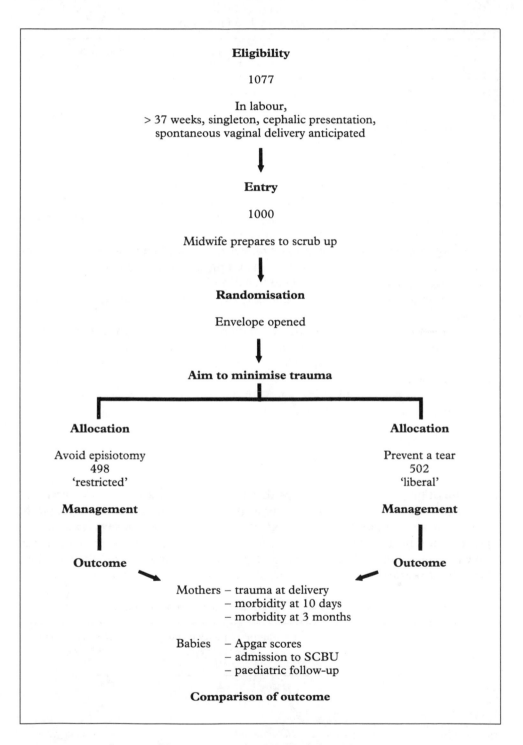

Fig. 2.1   Summary of the study design

Table 2.1   Descriptive data for entrants to trial

	Restricted policy group (n = 498)	Liberal policy group (n = 502)
Maternal age, mean (years)	26.6	26.7
Primiparous (%)	40	44
Married (%)	89	87
Gestational age, mean (weeks)	39.8	39.8
Birthweight, mean (g)	3393	3367

maternal age, parity and marital status. After delivery the midwives also noted the gestational age, Apgar score and birth weight of the babies. An assessment of perineal trauma, details of repair and the time taken to suture were documented by a doctor who was 'blind' to the trial allocation.

Ten days postpartum the community midwives assessed perineal healing and the mothers' reported residual problems, including persistent discomfort or pain. Standardised questionnaires were completed and returned via the internal mail. The community midwives were unaware of the trial allocation so bias was minimised.

Three months following delivery a postal questionnaire was sent to all participating mothers; a stamped, addressed envelope was enclosed for reply. A telephoned reminder was made to non-responders and a personal visit to those who did not have a telephone.

The response rate at both 10 days and 3 months postpartum was 89%, and there is no evidence that those lost to follow up differed between the two groups.

ANALYSIS AND RESULTS

Randomisation generated two groups that were similar in a number of important respects at trial entry (Table 2.1). The women were also delivered by people of comparable status (Table 2.2). Perineal trauma in the two groups was assessed by operators of similar experience (largely senior house officers) who were in ignorance of the trial allocation. It is worth considering what was being asked of the attendant midwives – to suspend their personal prejudices and, in the absence of foetal problems

Table 2.2   Status of persons performing deliveries

	Restricted policy group (n = 498) (%)	Liberal policy group (n = 502) (%)
Sister	33	31
Staff midwife	30	32
Student midwife	30	31
Medical student	5	5
Doctor	2	1

Table 2.3   Actual use of episiotomy

	Restricted policy group (n = 498) (%)	Liberal policy group (n = 502) (%)
Episiotomy rate	10.2	51.4
Primiparae	17.9	67.1
Multiparae	5.1	39.2
Maternal indications	3.6	45.4
Foetal distress	6.6	6.0

$\chi^2 = 196.37$ (1 d.f.), $p < 0.00001$

and the possibility of delivering without trauma to comply with a directive to withhold or perform an episiotomy. For many this meant a challenge to their most cherished beliefs.

The episiotomy rate was 10% in the group allocated to the restrictive policy and 51% in the liberal policy group (Table 2.3). The frequency of foetal indications for

Table 2.4   Maternal trauma at delivery

	Restricted policy group (n = 498) (%)	Liberal policy group (n = 502) (%)
Posterior trauma		
None	34	24
Episiotomy alone	9	45
Perineal tear alone	56	25
Episiotomy plus extension	1	6
Anterior trauma		
None	74	83
Labial tears	26	17

$\chi^2 = 11.29$ (1 d.f.), $p < 0.001$

episiotomy was similar in the two groups so the difference reflected the number of episiotomies performed for maternal reasons.

The different episiotomy rates resulted in differing patterns of trauma sustained at delivery. As anticipated, there were both more posterior tears and more intact

Table 2.5   Incidence of pain experienced by mothers at 10 days postpartum

Pain in last 24 hours	Restricted policy group (n = 439) (%)	Liberal policy group (n = 446) (%)
Mild	14.1	14.6
Moderate	7.5	7.8
Severe	0.9	0.2
Total	22.5	22.6

$\chi^2 = 1.91$ (3 d.f.), N.S.

Table 2.6   Incidence of pain experienced by mothers at 3 months postpartum

'Worst pain in last week'	Restricted policy group (n = 438) (%)	Liberal policy group (n = 457) (%)
Mild	4.6	5.7
Moderate	2.5	1.8
Severe	0.5	0.2
Total	7.6	7.7

$\chi^2 = 2.58$ (3 d.f.), N.S.

perinea among those allocated to the restricted policy (Table 2.4). There were also more anterior labial tears in this group. Severe maternal trauma was less common than anticipated. There were four cases in the restrictive and one in the liberal policy group.

Table 2.7   Time of resumption of sexual intercourse, investigated 3 months postpartum

	Restricted policy group (n = 438) (%)	Liberal policy group (n = 457) (%)
First month	37	27
Second month	44	53
Third month	10	10
Not yet	9	10

$p < 0.02$

There were no statistically significant differences in neonatal outcome. Despite the differing patterns and degrees of trauma the frequency of pain reported by mothers was very similar in the two groups both at 10 days after delivery (Table 2.5) and at 3 months postpartum (Table 2.6). Overall, 80% of women had resumed intercourse by the end of the second month following delivery and the numbers were the same in the two trial groups (Table 2.7). Within the first 4 weeks, however, those allocated to the restricted policy group were more likely to have resumed

Table 2.8   Involuntary loss of urine at 3 months postpartum

Do you ever lose any urine when you don't mean to?	Restricted policy group (n = 438) (%)	Liberal policy group (n = 457) (%)
No	81.1	81.0
Yes – no pad necessary	12.8	12.9
Yes – pad sometimes	5.9	5.3
Yes – pad always	0.2	0.7

N.S.

intercourse. This difference was only partly explained by the higher proportion of women with intact perinea. Of the women who had resumed intercourse, 52% in the restricted policy group and 51% in the liberal policy group had experienced dyspareunia at some time, and 22% and 18% respectively still had this problem 3 months postpartum.

Some degree of urinary incontinence was a common problem 3 months after delivery, but the different management policies appeared to have no effect on its reported frequency (Table 2.8).

DISCUSSION

This randomised controlled trial was designed to compare two policies for managing the perineum in spontaneous vaginal deliveries as they would be used in everyday midwifery practice. The study was conducted in a busy district hospital, and the deliveries were supervised by those who normally conducted spontaneous deliveries in the unit, 94% of whom were midwives.

Ninety-three per cent of eligible women were successfully recruited to the study, so the trial population may be considered to be representative of all non-instrumental deliveries during the 5-month period. There was good compliance with each of the trial directives, which was reflected in differing episiotomy rates in the two groups: 51% in the liberal policy group and 10% in the restricted policy group.

The only justification from this study for an episiotomy rate in excess of 10% in normal deliveries would be the possibility that the four cases of severe trauma in women allocated to the restricted policy could have been prevented. This difference may have been a real consequence of adopting a restrictive policy but it is possible that it could have been due to chance. This number was much lower than expected from other published studies. Overall, there was neither an increase nor a major decrease in the problems experienced by the mothers in the restrictive group in the 3 months following delivery; the only difference observed was a tendency for these women to resume sexual intercourse earlier. Overall, one in five women reported persistent dyspareunia at 3 months post-partum. The more restrictive policy resulted in substantial savings in suture materials. (If the results were extrapolated to the whole of England and Wales, the adoption of a restrictive policy would save an estimated £65,000-worth of suture material annually.) Although midwives took longer to deliver mothers when the use of episiotomy was restricted, this additional cost in midwifery time was of the same order as the increased medical staff time spent in suturing the additional trauma sites associated with the liberal policy.

Primiparae had more episiotomies, more anterior tears and fewer intact perinea than multiparae and they also sustained fewer posterior tears. Primiparae were also twice as likely to have pain at 10 days and at 3 months postpartum but were less likely to suffer involuntary loss of urine.

Nineteen per cent of mothers reported urinary incontinence 3 months after delivery, 6% of them needing to wear a pad for some or all of the time. There was no evidence that the liberal use of episiotomy prevented this problem.

These results of an experimental study that controlled for selection bias are in striking contrast with the findings of studies based on comparisons using observational data, all of which suggest that the discomfort after perineal tears is considerably less than after episiotomy. This highlights the importance of experimental design in evaluating different policies that govern care.

A follow-up of these mothers 3 years later has just been completed; this will assess the longer-term implications of the two policies in terms of maternal morbidity, especially urinary incontinence and vaginal prolapse. The findings are currently being analysed.

The results of this study suggest that the two currently opposing view points are both wrong. Tears do not appear to cause women fewer problems, neither do episiotomies result in better healing and improved recovery either in the short or long term. It is worth noting that restricting the operation resulted in 10% of mothers delivering with no trauma at all.

On the basis of these findings and in the absence of sound scientific evidence that this invasive, traumatic procedure is of positive benefit to a mother or her baby, the routine use of episiotomy should be discontinued. The procedure should only be used to relieve foetal distress or to progress delivery when it is the perineum that is responsible for lack of progress.

3 YEAR FOLLOW-UP STUDY

The women who participated in this study were recontacted by postal questionnaire 3 years after delivery (Sleep and Grant, 1987). This longer-term follow-up was designed to test the hypothesis that the liberal use of episiotomy protects against the subsequent development of urinary incontinence due to pelvic relaxation (Willson, 1981), but may be associated with an increased prevalence of dyspareunia (Kitzinger and Walters, 1981).

Table 2.9 Number (and percentage) of women with dyspareunia and urinary incontinence at 3 years post-partum

	Restrictive policy (n=329)	Liberal policy (n=345)
Ever suffering painful intercourse	52 (16)	45 (13)
With incontinence of urine:		
Once in past week	69 (22)	82 (25)
Once/twice in past week	37 (12)	35 (11)
Three or more times in past week	6 (2)	7 (2)
With incontinence sufficiently severe to wear a pad:		
Sometimes	26 (8)	24 (7)
Every day	5 (2)	4 (1)
With loss of urine:		
When coughing, laughing or sneezing	103 (33)	105 (31)
When urgent desire to pass urine but no toilet nearby	41 (13)	41 (13)

Altogether, 674 women out of the original sample of 1000 responded. There was no evidence of a differential response rate between the two trial groups. Pain during sexual intercourse and rates and severity of incontinence were almost identical in the two groups; this similarity persisted when deliveries in the intervening years were taken into account (Table 2.9). The liberal use of episiotomy does not, therefore, seem to prevent urinary incontinence or increase long-term dyspareunia. Some degree of stretching of the pelvic floor is inevitable during childbirth, but these findings support the results of other studies, which suggest that the function of pelvic floor muscles postnatally seems unrelated to perineal management at delivery (Gordon and Logue, 1985).

POSTSCRIPT

This experimental study has evaluated a clinical procedure that forms part of every-day midwifery care in the conduct of normal delivery. However, it raises several issues relating to perineal management, which have implications for women both during and after delivery.

On the tenth-day assessment form, mothers were invited to add comments in confidence. One of the most common criticisms was the inadequacy of analgesia prior to the performance of an episiotomy and before commencement of perineal repair. Both of these procedures are within the midwife's sphere of practice. In addition, the evidence of this study demonstrates that perineal pain in the early puerperium remains a major feature of maternal morbidity *whatever* the policy of perineal management at delivery. Primiparae are a particularly vulnerable group. These aspects of care form part of the midwife's responsibility, so it is important that she should be fully aware of these potential, treatable and largely preventable causes of maternal distress.

The data collected 3 months postpartum also provide midwives with an opportunity to appraise the longer-term implications of their management at a time when they no longer have contact with mothers. The reported frequencies of residual dyspareunia (20% overall) and urinary incontinence (affecting 19% of the women) raise issues regarding therapies that may be of use in the prevention or alleviation of these distressing symptoms, which have such a profound effect on the quality of life of the women for whom we care.

ACKNOWLEDGEMENTS

The trial was made possible by a large team of supportive and commited colleagues, principally: Dr Adrian Grant, who designed and supervised the trial, and his colleagues at the National Perinatal Epidemiology Unit (NPEU); Jo Garcia, who helped to design the questionnaires; Diana Elbourne, social statistician; and Iain Chalmers, Director of the unit. This study would not have been possible without their help, nor without the many midwives who worked so hard to make the trial such a success or John Spencer, Obstetric Registrar, who supervised the team of obstetricians. A special thank you must go to the mothers who responded so enthusiastically to requests for information about their experiences, and to Ann Medd for clerical assistance.

Jennifer Sleep was Maws Midwifery Scholar for 1982; additional funding for this project came from the locally organised (Oxford Region) research scheme. The NPEU was supported by a grant from the DHSS. A full report of this study was published by Sleep et al (1984).

REFERENCES

Cater, L. (1984) A little knowledge. *Nursing Mirror*, **159**(11): i–viii.

Chalmers, I. (1989) Evaluating the effects of care during pregnancy and childbirth. In: *Effective Care in Pregnancy and Childbirth*, Vol. 1, Chalmers, I., Enkin, M. and Kierse, M.J.N.C. (eds.), pp. 3–38. Oxford: Oxford University Press.

Donald, I. (1979) *Practical Obstetric Problems*. London: Lloyd-Luke.

Flood, C. (1982) The real reasons for performing episiotomies. *World Medicine*, Feb 6: 51.

Garcia, J., Garforth, S. and Ayres, S. (1985) Midwives confined? Labour ward policies and routines. In: *Research and the Midwife Conference Proceedings*, Thompson, A. and Robinson, S. (eds.), pp. 1–30. Nursing Research Unit, King's College, University of London.

Gordon, H. and Logue, M. (1985) Perineal muscle function after childbirth. *Lancet*, **ii**: 123–125.

Grant, A. (1982) Evaluating midwifery practice: the role of the randomised controlled trial. *Research and the Midwife Conference Proceedings*. Nursing Research Unit, King's College, University of London.

House, M.J. (1981) To do or not to do episiotomy. In *Episiotomy – Physical and Emotional Aspects*, Kitzinger, S. (ed.). London: National Childbirth Trust.

Kitzinger, S. and Walters, R. (1981) *Some Women's Experiences of Episiotomy*. London: National Childbirth Trust.

Macfarlane, A. and Mugford, M. (1984) *Birth Counts: Statistics of Pregnancy and Childbirth*. London: HMSO.

Sleep, J. and Grant, A. (1987) West Berkshire Perineal Management Trial: three year follow up. *British Medical Journal*, **295**: 749–751.

Sleep, J., Grant, A., Garcia, J., Elbourne, D., Spencer, J. and Chalmers, I. (1984) West Berkshire Perineal Management Trial. *British Medical Journal*, **289**: 587–590.

Thacker, S.B. and Banta, D. (1983) Benefits and risks of episiotomy: an interpretative review of the English language literature, 1860–1980. *Obstetric Gynaecological Survey*, **38**: 322–338.

Willson, J.R. (1982) Obstetrics–gynecology: a time for a change. *American Journal of Obstetrics and Gynecology*, **141**: 857–863.

Wilkerson, V.A. (1984) The use of episiotomy in normal delivery, *Midwives Chronicle and Nursing Notes*, **97**(1155): 106–110.

3

PAIN IN LABOUR

Kate Niven

'In sorrow thou shalt bring forth children' (Genesis iii, 16)

BACKGROUND TO THE STUDY

The study to be discussed forms part of a larger study of 'Factors affecting labour pain', details of which are published elsewhere (Niven and Gijsbers, 1984; Niven, 1985; Niven, 1986). The study as a whole was inspired by the possibility that psychological as well as physiological factors might influence the experience of labour pain. They, therefore, might contribute to the tremendous variability in the intensity of labour pain, which 'is too extensive to depend solely on the physiological factors involved' (Bonica, 1975).

Parturition is a complex physical, emotional and psychological event. Traditional theories of pain perception decree that any variation in the perception of pain must be due solely to variations in the amount of potentially tissue-damaging 'noxious' stimulation occurring (Von Frey, 1985). Thus, psychological and emotional factors, for example levels of anxiety, could have no part to play in exacerbating levels of pain. Modern pain theories (e.g. Melzack and Wall, 1988), in contrast, emphasise the role of psychological factors, interacting with physiological factors to modulate the experience of pain. Factors such as expectation, attention and emotional arousal are held to influence a person's experience of pain, and this proposition has been supported by the findings of clinical and experimental research. (For a general review of this research and of theories of pain the reader is directed to Melzack and Wall, 1988.)

Current theories of pain would predict that psychological factors could influence the perception of labour pain, but would not suggest that the degree of noxious stimulation caused by contraction of the uterus, dilation of the cervix, distention and traumatisation of the vagina and perineum is unimportant (Bonica, 1975). Thus any study of labour pain informed by these theories should concern itself with both psychological and physiological or obstetric factors. The study 'Factors affecting labour pain' included the consideration of a substantial number of psychological and physiological factors in relation to one another and also examined factors that are best defined as psycho-physiological, such as the one described in detail in this chapter, which involves the relationship between previous pain experience and labour pain experience.

The Previous Experience of Pain

Most instances of pain we suffer are coloured by our previous experiences of pain. Take for example, toothache. The first twinge, in my case, evokes horrific memories of sleepless nights, the smell of oil of cloves and the terror of the dentist's chair. Little wonder that my experience of toothache is exacerbated by my acute and illogical anxiety. For some more rational individuals the same first twinge evokes memories of quick, efficient and painless dental treatment and thus their twinge is less likely to become a raging toothache than mine. Other facets of previous pain experience may also influence my toothache, e.g. whether I have had a pain in the same tooth before, how I cope with toothache and how I cope with pain in general.

The effect of previous pain experience on current pain experience is considered important by many pain theorists today, but as yet only a limited amount of research, mainly on the effects of early pain experience, has been carried out. In this study the effect of all previous pain experience on the experience of pain in childbirth was examined. There were two broad hypotheses: first, that women who had suffered intense pain previously would experience more intense pain in childbirth than women whose previous pain experience had been more moderate; and, second, in direct opposition to the first, that women who had suffered intense pain previous to the current labour would suffer less pain during that birth than women who had had less pain in the past.

The rationale behind the first hypothesis was that women who had suffered intense pain in the past would be likely to suffer intense labour pain, since they were more sensitive to pain, had a lower threshold to pain or were more ready to complain of pain, than would subjects who reported a more moderate intensity of previous pain experience. There is evidence that sensitivity to pain is relatively stable over time (Hardy et al, 1952) as is the readiness to report pain (Sternbach, 1968), but such evidence has largely been gained from laboratory studies in which relatively low levels of pain are induced in subjects who know that there is no risk to 'life or limb' and that they can quit the experiment at any time. 'Real life' pain is very different, so similar stability may not be evident in this study, which concerns itself with real life experiences. A further criticism of this rationale is that the intensity of previous pain depends not only on a person's sensitivity to pain but also on the opportunities she has had to experience pain of high or low intensity. Has she given birth before? Is she involved in dangerous sports? Has she had serious illnesses or accidents? Such factors may be more crucial determinants of the intensity of previous pain than are threshold or complaint behaviour. However all parturants will have menstruated, and surely everybody has some aches and pains. The reported severity of these everyday pains may reflect stable individual differences in pain perception that will affect the perception of labour pain. This stability may be particularly noticeable when pain levels in a current labour are related to pain levels in a previous labour. Some obstetric factors such as the size and shape of the birth canal will not vary, and memories of an intensely painful or relatively painless previous birth will be especially salient to women during childbirth.

The second hypothesis is that the previous experience of intense pain will be related negatively, not positively, to levels of labour pain. Collins (1965) found that adult conscripts who had been very protected in childhood reported higher levels of experimentally induced pain than did those who had been more independent when young. The 'independent' group may have previously experienced more pain. Scott and Gijsbers (1981) found that among a group of competitive swimmers, those who had experienced more pain in training tolerated experimentally induced pain best. Furthermore, as training progressed, involving all the swimmers 'going through the pain barrier' regularly, their tolerance of pain increased. Both these studies suggest that the previous experience of pain may reduce the perception of subsequent pain under some circumstances. A similar effect may be found in labour, perhaps because intense pain is less frightening if it has been experienced, and survived, before, or because people learn to cope with intense pain through previous exposure to it.

METHOD

The main variables of interest in this study were the intensity of the subject's previous experience of pain and the intensity of labour pain in the subject's current birth.

Labour pain was assessed during the active phase of the first stage of labour and 24 to 48 hours postnatally, when subjects were required to recall the pain of both the first and second stages of labour. No attempt was made to assess pain during the second stage of labour since all the mother's energies at that time should be directed towards giving birth. Interfering with that process is unethical. Details of previous pain experience were obtained at the postnatal interview.

Two different assessment scales were used to record the subject's experience of labour pain: the McGill Pain Questionnaire (MPQ) and a Visual Analogue Scale (VAS). The MPQ makes use of words derived from those commonly used by physicians and patients to describe pain. The words have been assigned to 20 groups or categories based on statistically derived levels of agreement between subjects. These groups are considered to relate to three dimensions of pain – sensory, affective and evaluative – which reflect the complex neurological processes underlying pain perception. By attempting to reflect these different aspects of pain, the MPQ should provide data of a more subtle nature than those produced by simpler linear scales. The MPQ was used in this study to give detailed information on the nature and intensity of labour pain, a pain that has complex sensory and affective characteristics (Melzack and Wall, 1988). It is comparatively time-consuming to complete (although less than 5 minutes) and demands some competence in semantic comprehension. It might, therefore, be unsuitable for use with some labouring women. Accordingly, the VAS was used as an alternative and complementary method of pain assessment. It can be completed very quickly without resource to language.

The VAS (Scott and Huskisson, 1976) consists of a straight horizontal line, 10 cm long. The lower end point is labelled 'No pain' and the upper one 'Pain as bad as possible'. The subject is required to mark on the line the point that represents the intensity of the pain being assessed.

A substantial number of other variables was considered in the study as a whole, some of which might be related to the variables under discussion here. Information on variables such as parity was obtained from hospital records. Midwifery staff completed a questionnaire, which noted duration of labour, analgesic use, complications of birth, etc. The subject herself gave details of variables such as antenatal training and expectations of birth at the postnatal interview. These factors will only be discussed in this chapter if they relate to the variables under study.

SAMPLE SIZE AND CHARACTERISTICS

The subjects of this study were 101 British women giving birth in a modern, well-equipped and well-staffed maternity unit in central Scotland. Social classes II/III and IV/V were approximately equally represented. The women's age range was from 15 to 39 years, with an average age of 26. Four subjects were unmarried at the time of birth and had no current partner. Fifty-eight per cent of the sample were primiparous, 42% multiparous, 27% having their second baby, 12% their third and 1% each having their fourth, fifth and sixth child. Parturants who had severe anticipated foetal or maternal complications were excluded. Subjects who suffered from medical conditions unrelated to childbirth were not deliberately excluded but only one subject suffered from such a condition – rheumatoid arthritis. The subject population was, therefore, reasonably representative of the 'normal' British reproductive population.

'Abnormal' groups such as those at risk, the very young or old (in obstetric terms), the unhealthy and those from ethnic minorities were deliberately excluded from the sample because their inclusion would have necessitated the separate analysis of their data. The intended study of normal labour was complicated enough, involving overall an analysis of more than 100 variables. Subjects who were not native English speakers were excluded since the MPQ has not been validated for all other languages.

DATA COLLECTION

Data on labour pain was collected from the subjects during the first stage of labour and 24 to 48 hours after giving birth. All subjects who were in active labour – cervical dilation of at least 3 cm and a contraction rate of 2 in 10 min – during the investigator's afternoon visits were approached and, if informed consent was granted, completed the MPQ and VAS. The refusal rate was only 4%. Parturants who were receiving epidural anaesthesia, rarely used in the unit at the time of the study, were not included in this data collection, nor were parturants who were approaching transition.

The postnatal interview was carried out in the postnatal wards. The subjects again completed the MPQ and VAS to record their recall of the first and second stages of labour. They also answered a series of questions concerned with their previous experience of pain – 'What kind of pain?', 'How frequent was it?', 'How stressful?' – and they rated on the VAS the intensity of any previous labour pain and the most intense episode of previous pain unconnected with childbirth. This second

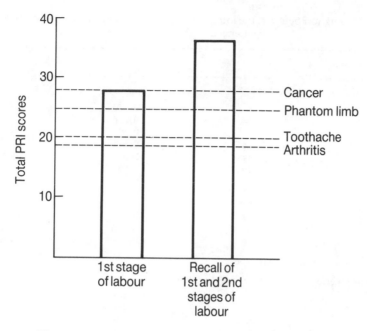

Fig. 3.1 Pain levels in labour (as assessed by the MPQ)

(Data on clinical disorders from Melzack, 1975)

interview was sometimes interrupted by the baby's or the staff's needs. Consequently, some interviews were incomplete and the number of sets of data obtained in this interview was often less than for first interview.

ANALYSIS AND RESULTS

The MPQ yielded data on the intensity of the sensory, affective and evaluative dimensions of labour pain, a Total Pain Ranking Index (Total PRI) and a five-point assessment of Present Pain Intensity (PPI). The VAS was scored from 0 to 10. Labour pain scores recorded during the first stage of labour are categorised as Sensory 1, VA 1, etc. Recall scores recorded during the second interview are categorised as Sensory 2, etc. All data were analysed using parametric statistics.

The average intensity of labour pain was severe (Figure 3.1) but varied considerably. For instance, first stage scores on the VAS ranged from 0 to 9.5, and VA 2 scores from 1.5 to 10. As 0 represents 'no pain' and 10 pain 'as bad as possible', it can be seen that the variation was extreme. Some of that variability was related to previous pain experience. There was a positive correlation between the intensity of pain experienced in the current birth and the intensity of pain in previous births. As can be seen in Table 3.1, the levels of correlation were high enough on a number of pain measures to be statistically significant and were, therefore, unlikely to be merely due to chance. However, they were not high enough to suggest that a woman who has a painful birth on one occasion will invariably have painful births again.

Table 3.1   Correlation between the intensity of pain experienced in previous births and that experienced in the current birth

Labour pain measure	n	r	p
Subjects who had only one previous birth			
Sensory 1	34	0.140	N.S.
Affective 1	34	0.116	N.S.
Evaluative 1	34	0.007	N.S.
Total PRI 1	34	0.141	N.S.
PPI 1	34	0.126	N.S.
VA 1	25	−0.156	N.S.
Sensory 2	34	0.297	<0.1
Affective 2	34	0.334	$<0.05\star$
Evaluative 2	34	0.496	$<0.01\star\star$
Total PRI 2	34	0.376	$<0.05\star$
PPI 2	34	0.420	$<0.01\star\star$
VA 2	26	0.273	N.S.
Subjects who had two or more previous births			
(Correlations reported are only those that were significant)			
Sensory 1	17	0.498	$<0.05\star$
Total PRI 1	17	0.450	<0.1
Sensory 2	15	0.605	$<0.01\star$
PPI 2	15	0.566	$<0.02\star$
VA 2	12	0.656	$<0.02\star$

N.S. = Not significant
$\star$ $= p < 0.05$
$\star\star = p < 0.01$

Correlations between the intensity of previous pain unconnected with childbirth and the intensity of labour pain (current) were very low and non-significant, e.g. Total PRI 1, $r = -0.02$; Total PRI 2, $r = 0.04$. This was because the relationship between the two variables was complex.

In order to clarify the relationship the data were divided in two ways. First, data from primiparae were analysed separately from data for multiparae, as parity was independently related to differences in levels of labour pain (Niven and Gijsbers, 1984) so may have confounded the relationship between previous pain and labour pain. Second, previous pain experience was split into three groups – no previous pain (NPP), low previous pain (LPP) and high previous pain (HPP). Subjects were assigned to one of these three groups according to their assessment of the intensity of previous pain on the VAS. If subjects maintained, despite careful probing, that they had never experienced pain outside childbirth, they were categorised as NPP. LPP subjects had assessed their previous pain as less than 6 on the VAS, HPP subjects as more than 6. The split point of 6 was used as it was the median score.

Figure 3.2 shows the levels of labour pain experienced for these three groups. NPP subjects had the lowest levels of labour pain. HPP subjects had lower levels of labour pain than did LPP subjects, particularly if they were primiparous. An analysis of variance and individual t tests were carried out, which confirmed these findings (Tables 3.2 and 3.3, below). A check was made to see if any variable that was

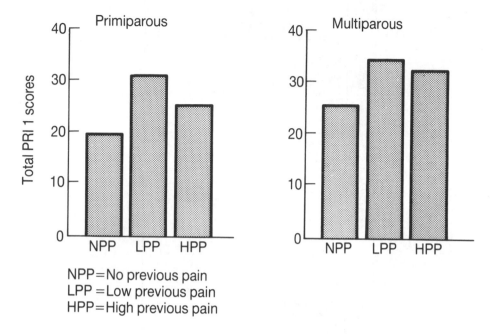

NPP=No previous pain
LPP =Low previous pain
HPP=High previous pain

Fig. 3.2   The relationship between the intensity of previous pain unrelated to childbirth and
levels of labour pain in primiparae and multiparae

associated with significant differences in labour pain was also associated with the
groupings of previous pain experience. Analgesic use was marginally associated with
previous pain experience. In order to control for its effects statistically, an analysis of
co-variance was carried out, which improved the significance of the findings. This
established that the relationship between previous pain experience and labour pain
experience was not due to the effects of differential analgesic use. These findings are
summarised in Table 3.3.

The most common type of pain suffered by the subjects was dysmenorrhoea.
Other common pains were headaches and back pain. A few subjects had experienced intense pain associated with surgery or trauma. These unusual experiences
may have influenced the findings. Accordingly, the data on dysmenorrhoea, a type
of pain that all subjects *could* have suffered, were analysed separately. The results
followed the same pattern as the findings already described. Subjects who had
suffered intense dysmenorrhoea had significantly lower levels of labour pain than
those who had suffered more moderate pain ($F = 4.19$, d.f.1.25, $p < 0.05$).

The results of this study can, therefore, be summarised as follows:

1. There was a positive correlation between the intensity of pain in previous
births and the intensity of pain in the current birth.
2. Primiparous and multiparous subjects who had never experienced pain unconnected with childbirth had the lowest levels of pain in labour.
3. Primiparae who had experienced severe pain previously had significantly lower
levels of labour pain than those who had previously experienced less intense

Table 3.2 Levels of labour pain and the intensity of previous pain

Labour pain measurement	n	NPP	S.D.	n	LPP	S.D.	n	HPP	S.D.	F	p
Primiparae											
Sensory 1	6	15.6	4.8	26	23.6	8.0	26	18.8	6.2	4.76	0.01**
Affective 1	6	2.5	4.2	26	5.4	4.1	26	4.0	3.4	1.83	0.17
Evaluative 1	6	1.3	1.3	26	2.6	1.5	26	2.4	1.7	1.64	0.20
Total PRI 1	6	19.5	7.8	26	31.8	11.6	26	25.2	9.3	4.68	0.01**
PPI 1	6	2.1	0.4	25	2.8	1.1	22	2.5	1.0	1.10	0.34
VA 1	4	6.7	2.4	21	5.5	2.6	22	5.6	2.3	0.39	0.67
Sensory 2	5	16.0	9.8	24	28.5	11.2	26	21.4	7.7	5.41	0.007**
Affective 2	5	4.6	5.3	24	7.5	3.9	26	5.6	3.1	2.23	0.11
Evaluative 2	5	2.6	2.4	24	3.4	1.4	26	3.3	1.7	0.50	0.60
Total PRI 2	5	23.2	17.1	24	39.1	15.0	26	29.8	10.7	4.57	0.01**
PRI 2	5	2.0	0.7	24	3.1	1.0	25	3.0	1.1	2.27	0.11
VA 2	3	7.5	2.1	22	7.6	2.0	25	8.2	1.5	0.85	0.43
*Multiparae**											
PPI 2	4	8.7	0.7	14	7.7	1.6	15	8.0	2.1	0.32	0.73

NPP = No previous pain
LPP = Low previous pain
HPP = High previous pain
* = Only significant data are given
** = p <0.01

Table 3.3 Significant differences in labour pain levels for subjects with differing intensities of previous pain

Primiparae only

Labour pain measure	Previous pain groups	t	p	Co-variant† t	Co-variant† p
Sensory 1	NPP/LPP	2.51	0.01	2.80	0.007*
Sensory 1	LPP/HPP	2.48	0.01	3.02	0.003*
Total PRI 1	NPP/LPP	2.63	0.01	2.73	0.008*
	LPP/HPP	2.29	0.02	3.05	0.003*
Sensory 2	NPP/LPP	2.67	0.01	3.03	0.003*
Sensory 2	LPP/HPP	2.63	0.01	2.98	0.004*
Total PRI 2	NPP/LPP	2.43	0.01	2.68	0.009*
	LPP/HPP	2.45	0.01	2.78	0.007*

Multiparae only

Labour pain measure	Previous pain groups	t	p	Co-variant† t	Co-variant† p
PPI 2	NPP/LPP	-2.54	0.01	-2.68	0.009*

† Pethidine and Entonox as co-variants
* Significant level on Bonferonni test

NPP = No previous pain
LPP = Low previous pain
HPP = High previous pain

pain. The relationship in multiparae was similar but was not strong enough to be significant.

4. Subjects who had had severe dysmenorrhoea had lower levels of labour pain than subjects who had experienced less intense period pain.

DISCUSSION

The results of this study suggest that the intensity of labour pain is related to previous pain experiences. The nature of that relationship is complex, its direction depending on the kind of pain involved – whether or not it is associated with childbirth – and on its intensity. These factors are best discussed separately at first.

Previous Labour Pain

Many midwives concerned with predicting how much pain their patient will have in labour ask multiparae how much pain they had in their previous births. The usefulness of this 'rule of thumb' is borne out by the results of this study. The positive correlations found between the intensity of pain in successive labours should not be taken to imply that women suffer the *same* amount of pain in subsequent births, but that those who suffered little in a previous birth are likely to suffer less in a current birth than are those who suffered severely before. This tendency is likely to be due to the stability of factors such as the size and shape of the birth canal, the distribution of relevant receptors, etc. It may be affected by factors that interfere with that stability, for example the size and position of the baby. The evidence of this study on the effects of previous pain experience unrelated to childbirth suggests that this factor, too, may moderate this tendency to some extent (see Figure 3.2, above).

Previous Pain Unrelated to Childbirth

NPP Subjects

This small and unusual group of subjects experienced the lowest levels of labour pain. It is unlikely that they had forgotten or were lying about some previous pain experience since their lack of pain was probed very thoroughly by the interviewer. Their responses probably accurately reflected their relative insensitivity to pain, an insensitivity that meant that they only experienced pain when exposed to intense stimulation, as in childbirth.

Unless the subject population of this study was grossly unrepresentative of the reproductive population as a whole, a similarly reduced sensitivity to noxious stimulation must exist in about 10% of all parturants. Although cases of total insensitivity to pain, associated with mental deficiency, unrecognised injury and early death, have been recorded (see Melzack and Wall, 1988) no recognition of a group such as this one is apparent from a cursory search of the medical and obstetric literature.

The results of this study suggest that formal recognition of this group would be useful since it is likely that they will not suffer intense pain in labour (Niven and Gijsbers, in press).

LPP and HPP Subjects

These subjects were in the majority. Their range of pain experience was quite extensive, from mild dysmenorrhoea (VAS = 2) to intense prolonged pain following thoracic surgery (VAS = 10). Those subjects who had experienced severe pain in the past had lower levels of labour pain than those whose previous pain experience had been more moderate. This inverse relationship between the intensity of previous pain and the intensity of labour pain was strongest in primiparae, which was not surprising, most multiparae having suffered severe pain in the past – in labour.

This result is somewhat against intuition, although supported by the findings of Collins (1965) and Scott and Gijsbers (1981). Is it perhaps a spurious result, produced by some association with another variable or by some anomaly in the pain assessment procedure? The only variable that was clearly associated with differences in previous pain experience and independently associated with levels of labour pain was analgesic use. Statistical control of the effects of analgesic use improved the relationship between previous pain experience and levels of labour pain, so this relationship was not due to the effects of pethidine and Entonox.

Subjects were required to assess the intensity of previous pain and the intensity of labour pain (by recall) at the same (the postnatal) interview. This requirement could have encouraged contrast effects in these assessments. Such effects would arguably be most evident on the VAS, since the VAS was common to both assessments, and on the data obtained in the postnatal interview, and not during labour when previous pain had not been considered. The results in Table 3.2 above show that there was no contrast between VAS assessments (a high score on one was not offset by a low score on the other) and that there were significant differences in labour pain levels for LPP and HPP subjects recorded during labour as well as postnatally. Furthermore, the results of a separate study (Gijsbers and Niven, in press) showed that subjects did not change their assessment of the intensity of previous pain after giving birth. So it seems that subjects do not exaggerate or minimise their rating of previous pain intensity when comparing it with their rating of labour pain.

The same inverse relationship between the intensity of previous pain and levels of labour pain was found when the type of pain involved was restricted to dysmenorrhoea and, in another part of the study, when previous pain experience was assessed by independent raters rather than by the subject (Niven, 1986). Furthermore, Rivière and Chastrusse (1954) made a similar observation in dogs, noting that bitches who had a rough upbringing showed less discomfort whelping than did bitches more gently reared. It seems, therefore, that the relationship between the previous experience of intense pain and lower levels of pain in labour is not spurious. What can explain it?

Scott and Gijsbers (1981) suggest that some short-term neurohormonal adaptation to pain might have operated in their swimmers. The operation of such a mechanism could not explain the effects of intense pain occurring many years before, although some long-term neurohormonal changes cannot be ruled out. The experience of intense pain has obvious psychological consequences, however, and these might explain the relationship.

If one suffers intense pain and survives it, one must learn something from that experience, perhaps to cope with severe pain or perhaps just that it can be lived through, something that women in labour have been known to doubt! Either way, the woman who has suffered severe pain in the past could be in a better position to cope with the intense pain of labour than is the woman who has experienced nothing more traumatic than a mild headache.

This possibility was explored in a study of the subjects' coping behaviour (Niven and Gijsbers, in press), which cannot be detailed here because of lack of space. Its results can be summarised as showing that women who have suffered severe pain in the past:

1. use more psychological coping strategies when in pain;
2. use more coping strategies when in labour;
3. use more of the same coping strategies in labour that they used when previously suffering pain.

These findings, which were statistically significant, suggest that women who have experienced severe pain in the past have learned how to cope with such pain through the use of strategies such as relaxation or distraction. Their expertise in the implementation of these strategies is then put to use in coping with labour pain.

Empirical studies have shown that the use of psychological strategies reduces levels of pain (see Melzack and Wall [1988] for a review of these studies). Presumably, the use of familiar, well-rehearsed strategies during labour by women who have used them previously to cope with intense pain results in some reduction in labour pain and goes some way to explaining the lower levels of pain found in HPP subjects. Other psychological factors are probably also involved, for example less fear of pain. Rivière and Chastrusse's observations suggest that more basic, non-psychological mechanisms may operate as well, since it is unlikely that dogs use psychological coping strategies!

CONCLUSION

A woman's previous experience of pain is likely to affect her experience of labour pain. If she has given birth before, the amount of pain she experienced in the previous birth gives some indication of how much pain she will suffer in the current birth, particularly if she suffered little pain during labour and no pain outside childbirth.

A small number of primiparous women may never have suffered pain before going into labour. They are likely to suffer comparatively mild pain in labour. However, the experience of pain will be new to them, so may be especially alarming. Their experience should, therefore, not be trivialised. Most primiparae will have experienced pain before. The results of this study suggest that those who have previously suffered intense pain will have less pain in labour than those who have suffered less severely in the past. This may be because they have learned to cope more effectively with intense pain:

Suffering passes but the fact of having suffered never passes. (Bloy, 1961)

ACKNOWLEDGEMENTS

The author would like to thank Dr K. Gijsbers, Department of Psychology, Stirling University, for his supervision of the thesis of which this study forms a part, Dr K. Stewart, Miss M. Forrest and their staff at Stirling Royal Infirmary Maternity Unit for their co-operation with the data collection, and the Nuffield Foundation for their financial support.

REFERENCES

Bonica, J.J. (1975) The nature of pain of parturition. In: *Obstetric Analgesia and Anaesthesia: Recent Advances and Current States*, Bonica, J.J. (ed.). New York: W B Saunders.

Bloy, L. (1961) Le pelerin de l'absolu. In: *Pain*, Buytendijk, F.J.J. (ed.). London: Hutcheson.

Collins, L.G. (1965) Pain sensitivity and ratings of childhood experience. *Perceptual and Motor Skills*, 21: 349–350.

Hardy, J., Wolff, H. and Goodell, H. (1952) *Pain Sensations and Reactions*. Baltimore: Williams and Wilkins.

Melzack, R. (1975) The McGill Pain Questionnaire: major properties and scoring methods. *Pain*, 1: 277–299.

Melzack, R. and Wall, P.D. (1988) *The Challenge of Pain*, 2nd edn. Harmondsworth: Penguin.

Niven, C. (1985) How helpful is the presence of the husband at childbirth? *Journal of Reproductive and Infant Psychology*, 3: 45–53.

Niven, C. (1986) *Factors Affecting Labour Pain*. Unpublished PhD thesis, University of Stirling.

Niven, C. and Gijsbers, K. (1984) Obstetric and non-obstetric factors related to labour pain. *Journal of Reproductive and Infant Psychology*, 2: 61–78.

Niven, C. and Gijsbers, K. Low levels of labour pain: an example of unusually low sensitivity to noxious stimulation? *Pain*, in press.

Rivière, M. and Chastrusse, L. (1954) La douleur en obstétrique. *Revue Français de Gynécologie et D'obstétrique*, 49: 247–276.

Scott, V. and Gijsbers, K. (1981) Pain perception in competitive swimmers. *British Medical Journal*, 283: 91–93.

Scott, J. and Huskisson, E.C. (1976) Graphic representation of pain. *Pain*, 2: 175–184.

Sternbach, R.A. (1968) *Pain: A Psychophysiological Analysis*. New York: Academic Press.

Von Frey, M. (1895) Bietrage zur Sinnesphysiologie der Haut. *Ber. d. kgl. sachs. Ges. d. Wiss. Math.-phys. Ke.*, 47: 166–184.

4

PSYCHOLOGICAL INSIGHTS INTO EARLY FEEDING EXPERIENCE

Peter Wright

At first glance a midwife might well raise her eyebrows as to why a psychologist should be writing about feeding in infancy, as she will probably share the lay person's view that a psychologist is only concerned with unconscious wishes and abnormal behaviour. It is, therefore, worthwhile at the start of this chapter making clear that a psychologist is interested in all aspects of human behaviour and that this will include the origins and development of that behaviour. Indeed, the topic of motivation that subsumes the classic primary drives of hunger and thirst has a long and detailed history and has in recent years been especially influenced by ideas from the discipline of ethology, which seeks to describe the behaviour of organisms in their natural conditions. Ethologists often rely on observational techniques in which detailed records of the behaviours shown by the animal in the period of observation are taken. Essentially the same approach is often used with young infants, and at one level it is exactly what any mother tries to do when she observes her baby and attempts to make sense of the behaviour or, more often, tries to detect a pattern of meaning in that behaviour.

Although the midwife is predominantly concerned with infant feeding in the immediate neonatal period, she also needs to be aware of the subsequent changes in feeding behaviour that will occur as the baby develops. One major reason for this is that she may then be in a position to help the very large group of mothers who begin breast feeding but who terminate the process fairly rapidly within a few weeks of birth. Despite the effort and research that have been directed at antenatal education to encourage and prepare women to breast feed, scant attention has been paid to the need for continued or extended education in the immediate postnatal period. At this stage, in the first few days after birth, the decision to breast feed has already been taken, and the realities and problems of breast feeding are confronting the mother. There is (at least for first-time mothers) a 'captive audience' in the wards and some breast-feeding mothers will have had little or no education antenatally: attendance at antenatal classes ranges from 30–50% and many do not complete the full course (Black et al, 1984).

The national policy is to encourage mothers to fully breast feed until the baby is 3 to 4 months old. Whereas there is universal encouragement of this policy on the wards, the indications are that although large numbers of mothers may breast feed when in hospital, one third of those who were breast feeding in hospital will have given up by 6 weeks after delivery (DHSS, 1980; Martin and White, 1988; DHSS, 1989). This was found to be the case in Edinburgh (Wright, 1981; Wright and Crow, 1982) and there are a number of reasons for this pattern. Some mothers will conform to the ward pressure to breast feed but will revert to the bottle almost immediately. Other mothers will abandon breast feeding at some stage within the first 6 weeks owing to problems for which they are unprepared, both in knowledge and expectation.

Yet, despite some considerable improvement in recent years in the proportion of women who commence breast feeding in hospital (Martin and Monk, 1982), survey after survey reports a dramatic drop in proportion in the few weeks after leaving hospital. The results of a recent (unpublished) Edinburgh survey are shown in Figure 4.1, as a survivorship analysis, which is a technique widely used in medical research, for example in studies of treatment outcomes. In this particular instance, a logarithmic scale has been used to make the picture more clear. There is a break in the curve at around 6 weeks of age and, clearly, we are looking at two different populations. The slope of the line shows that the probability that mothers will terminate breast feeding is high in the first 6 weeks. At around the 6-week point, however, there is an abrupt change in the slope and this shows that the mothers who 'survive' into the period beyond 6 weeks are much less likely to give up. Six weeks, then, is a critical point or hurdle, which, if surmounted, means that a mother is likely to continue to fully breast feed for the recommended period.

SUCCESSFUL AND UNSUCCESSFUL BREAST FEEDING

What are the differences between the unsuccessful and the successful breast-feeding groups? No difference could be found in the reasons they gave for wanting to breast

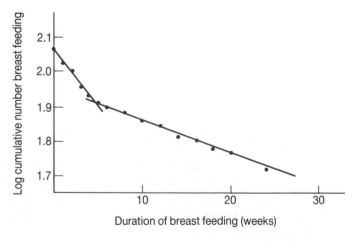

Fig 4.1   Log Survivorship plot of breast feeding duration

feed in the first place, with both being equally positive about the perceived benefits of breast feeding. When the reasons given for terminating breast feeding were examined, the majority of our sample, apart from a few who considered 6 weeks to be 'successful' and had never intended to feed any longer than this, produced the usual wide variety of reasons, in which the claim to have insufficient milk was by far the most common. Because so many studies have the same finding (Sacks et al, 1976; West, 1980; Martin and Monk, 1982) there is the very real possibility that the belief becomes common knowledge in the community, and that despite their knowledge of the physiology of lactation, many nurses may have the sneaking suspicion that it is also true.

In discussing survey results almost identical to the above, McIntosh (1985) comments that 71% of his sample stopped breast feeding for physical and not social reasons, with insufficient milk being reported by half the mothers. It has been suggested (Newson and Newson, 1963) that physical reasons are put forward by women who have underlying social objections to breast feeding or who have reluctantly felt obliged to go through the motions of attempting to breast feed. McIntosh argues that such physical claims are likely to be genuine on the grounds that those who firmly oppose breast feeding do not attempt it in the first place but, more importantly, because of the spontaneous and clearly genuine expression of disappointment and regret at their failure.

In order to prepare for problems that may be encountered by the mothers, we need to have a firm understanding of how feeding changes over time. Feeding during the first week of life is going to be a very different experience for both infant and mother than it will be once lactation is firmly established, and it is important for the mother to realise that the behaviour of her infant may differ in characteristic ways from that of the bottle-fed baby in the next cot. Mothers inevitably make such comparisons and will continue to do so as they visit postnatal clinics and discuss their experiences with their contemporaries. Some of these differences between the bottle-fed and the breast-fed baby are described elsewhere (Wright et al, 1980; Wright, 1988). Suffice it to mention here that in the first week breast-fed infants appear more hungry than those bottle fed (Richards and Bernal, 1972) and, of course, in these first few days the 24-hour intake of bottle-fed infants is constant, whereas the breast-fed infant experiences a gradual increase in intake from day to day. Bottle-fed babies consume more food on the third day of life than do breast-fed babies, and in a biological sense can be said to have consumed too much. It was also apparent that if bottle-fed babies were fed frequently, they consumed the same amount at each feed as those fed less frequently, whereas the breast-fed babies appeared to regulate their intake and took less at each feed the more frequently they fed. It was also found that at 3 to 4 days of age babies do not sleep longer if they have a larger meal (Crow and Wright, 1976). One implication of this is that during very early infancy one cannot guarantee a peaceful night for the mother by giving the baby an extra ounce of milk. Another interesting example in which the infant's behaviour and the mother's beliefs do not match comes from asking mothers whether they thought babies slept longer after a large meal: both breast- and bottle-feeding mothers tended to agree that they did (Table 4.1).

Table 4.1   Do babies sleep longer following a large meal?

	Breast		Bottle	
	Yes	No	Yes	No
1–2 weeks	17	4	24	2
2–4 months	14	8	20	0

THE MOTHER'S CONCEPT OF FEEDING

In earlier studies (Crow and Wright, 1976; Crow, 1977) a large sample of mothers was asked a number of open-ended questions designed to reveal their knowledge about infant feeding. The responses for two of these questions from the first 50 breast feeders and 50 bottle feeders have been used to illustrate the nature of the replies, and as the answers have been selected from a wider set of responses, no statistical analysis has been made. The results are reported here to show the value of this kind of interview in providing some insight into the context in which feeding occurs.

Question 1: What Aspects Do You Consider To Be Important To Pay Attention To When Feeding Your Baby?

Replies to this question fell into three categories: baby-directed activities, technical aspects of feeding practice and concern with what might be called the psychological environment. Baby-directed activities included the expressed need for mother to look at, talk to and cuddle the baby; the technical aspects of feeding practice included care that the baby was fixed at the breast, that the food was warm, that the baby was properly winded and that the constituents of the food were correct; whereas the psychological environment concerned the need for mother and baby to be relaxed and to enjoy the feed.

The findings are interesting. Although mothers gave more than one example in their replies, the number of responses given showed that both breast- and bottle-feeding mothers considered it important to interact with the baby (15 positive responses by breast feeders compared to 14 by bottle feeders) and to make sure that the technical aspects of the feed were satisfactory (56 positive responses by breast feeders and 39 by bottle feeders). Where the two groups differed was in their concern regarding the psychological environment. It seemed considerably more important to the breast-feeding mothers that *both* mother and baby enjoyed the feed in a relaxed atmosphere (76 positive responses compared to 6).

This need not, of course, mean that bottle-feeding mothers ignored this aspect, but rather, it might be said, that it was not a preoccupation of theirs. Why this difference? Is it because in encouraging mothers to breast feed, midwives and health visitors stress these aspects? Or is it something that mothers have read about in the lay literature? It is certainly a finding that may have important implications for practice since, if this is an expectation of how breast feeding should be experienced, does it in fact reflect reality?

On several occasions mothers who were breast feeding commented that it was a pity that no-one had warned them that they might feel tired or even uncomfortable when feeding. It is, therefore, possible that failure to teach such expectations could influence a mother's relationship with her baby and jeopardise the successful outcome of breast feeding (Wright, 1987b).

Question 2: What Criteria Do You Use To Decide That The Baby Has Had Enough?

The criteria used by mothers were: 'Baby stops sucking', 'Baby is sleepy', 'Baby looks content', 'Baby spits out the teat/nipple' and 'According to the advice offered by the nurse'. The differences in response that emerge from the answers given to this question are that whereas more breast-feeding than bottle-feeding mothers recognise falling asleep as a satiety cue (21 responses from breast feeders and 3 from bottle feeders), more bottle-feeding mothers stop feeding only when the baby spits out the teat (16 responses from bottle feeders and 2 from breast feeders). This finding becomes more interesting when considered in relation to direct observations of infant feeding behaviour (Wright et al, 1980). There seem to be several stages in the process of terminating a feed – the baby slows down its suck rate, becomes drowsy and, if mother still continues to feed, will refuse to open its mouth or will spit out the teat if it is forced into the mouth. In terms of this progression it would appear that some bottle-feeding mothers are more likely to override the early signs of satiety and are thus in greater danger of overfeeding their baby. Interpreted in these terms, this finding would be an example of an environmental factor that could contribute to the development of rapid weight gain and obesity (Wright, 1981).

DEVELOPMENTAL STUDIES OF INFANT FEEDING

The observational techniques referred to at the beginning of this chapter were used to videotape mothers feeding their babies at all ages from birth until 6 months of age. Subsequent analysis of the tapes enabled description of the kinds of interaction that occur during the course of the feed.

Feeds are continuously interrupted by removal of the bottle or breast for a variety of reasons – choking, winding the baby, possetting of food, changing breast, etc. – and from the videotaped records each interruption was scored in terms of whether it was baby or mother determined (Figure 4.2). Such interruptions in the case of bottle-fed babies are almost entirely under the control of the mother. On the other hand, among breast-fed babies some interruptions are determined by the mother, but more by the baby. These results are in agreement with others for the 1-week-old infant (Dunn, 1975) and indicate that although inexperience on the part of the mother could account for such interruptions at 1 week of age, the behaviour becomes established and is consistent across all three ages. A further consequence of the dominant mother control in the bottle-fed baby is that the pattern of the feed is sometimes disrupted when the baby is stimulated by the mother into resuming

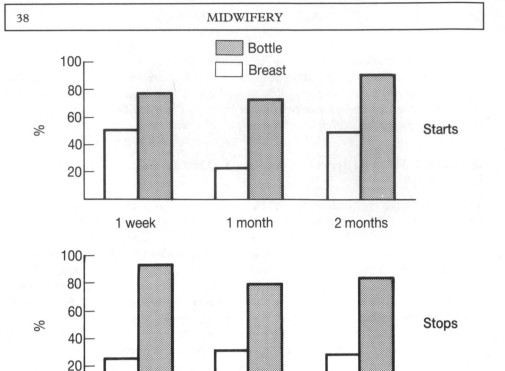

Fig 4.2   Analysis of teat or nipple in/out behaviour throughout videotaped feeds, expressed as a percentage of the number of occasions when the mother was the initiator of the behaviour

sucking, so the breast-fed baby has a greater opportunity to determine the pace and duration of its feeds.

MEAL PATTERNS IN THE FIRST WEEKS

Because of interest in the regulation of food intake and how this develops in infancy, mothers were asked to provide a detailed record of their baby's intake for a few days each month. One of the aims here was to see how much individual variation there is in the intake and growth of the babies. It is now a standard practice of many GPs and health visitors to provide a mother with growth charts on which she can plot her own infant's weight gain. A problem with this practice is that she may become concerned at a falling rate of gain compared to the chart and start solids or even stop breast feeding. As Paul and Whitehead (1986) have previously pointed out, we still do not know enough to make a decision over whether to base targets for the infant growth rate on the breast-fed baby, particularly as the late introduction of solids is normal. More data are needed on the growth of breast-fed babies so that adequate growth charts can be constructed and a more realistic interpretation of growth obtained.

Mothers are recruited into the study either through local health centres or through the National Childbirth Trust. Mothers have to be relied on for collecting and accurately reporting their own data in this kind of project, and because the object of the research is clearly of great interest to them, their records have been found to be detailed and highly reliable. One particular interest of the research is the relationship between the mother's perception of how hungry her infant was at a particular feed and the actual milk intake. The mothers have the aims of the study explained to them and they are provided with a digital electronic balance, which gives an accurate and instant weight for the baby, compensating for body movements while the weight is being taken. The protocol left with the mother contains the following instructions:

> 'We would like you to enter all occasions when you feed your infant over the next 4 consecutive days, but we don't always expect you to achieve this! If you forget, or baby makes things difficult, just mention what happened on the sheet; the important thing is that we should know when the meals occurred. As we are particularly interested in how much breast milk your baby takes at each feed, we want you to weigh the baby on the scales immediately before and immediately after the feed. It is important that you do not change the baby's clothing in between the two weighings as the difference between the two weighings is a measure of how much breast milk has been taken. When you decide to feed, note the time of day (indicate whether it is a.m. or p.m.) and weigh the baby. At the end of the feed and *before* you weigh baby again, mark on the line how hungry you feel your baby was at that feed. You should feel free to use the whole of the scale provided. Then weigh the baby again and record the time at which the feed ends.

Example:

> Not at all hungry --------------------------------- X ----------- Very hungry indeed

This position might follow a feed where there were few problems, baby seemed very hungry and you felt that baby was satisfied at the end of the feed.

Example:

> Not at all hungry ---------------------- X ---------------------- Very hungry indeed

This could be an average feed, not filled with crying episodes and bringing up milk, but neither did you feel baby had taken much or enjoyed the feed as much as others you had given.'

Before the mother starts to keep one of these records, she is asked a series of informal questions, which include:

1. Do you think your baby is more hungry or less hungry at any particular time in the course of a 24-hour day?
2. What makes you think he or she is more or less hungry at this time?
3. Do you feel your own supply of breast milk is less at any stage in the 24 hours?

Quite deliberately, no attempt is made to define hunger as the interest lies in the kinds of event and behaviour that mothers attribute to hunger.

RESULTS

Figure 4.3 plots the mean meal size across the 24-hour period. The mean meal size is obtained by grouping together all the meals that fall into a single-4 hour period;

for example, if a meal was initiated between midnight and 4 a.m., it would contribute to the mean meal size plotted for 2 a.m., and so on for 6 a.m., 10 a.m., etc. It does not indicate a group of clockwork mothers all feeding at exactly 4-hourly intervals! When the babies are 1 week old and even 1 month old, there is no difference in the size of these meals across the 24 hours, but by the age of 8 weeks all the infants have established a very clear diurnal pattern of responding with the largest meal falling between 4 a.m. and 8 a.m. and meals then becoming progressively smaller throughout the day. Exactly this same pattern has been found in several repeats of the original study. At some point between 5 and 7 weeks of age, the meal size pattern shifts from equal feeds to this large meal in the morning, often when the baby has begun to drop the meal that would have fallen in the very early hours of the morning.

In older infants who continue to be breast fed, the pattern changes again, so that between 4 and 6 months of age the smallest meals of the day occur first thing in the morning and the largest meals at the end of the day (Wright and Crow, 1982). This may represent a switch from a more primitive form of responding characterised as *deficit responding*, i.e. large meals follow long intervals without food, to *anticipatory responding* in the older infant, with large meals now being taken before the overnight feed. This change is speculated to be a learned pattern on the part of the infant rather than a passive response to, for instance, changes in the composition of the breast milk with time of day or age. This latter belief that the milk intake of breast-fed infants is influenced by changes in the fat content of the fore and hind milk, although an attractive and widely quoted hypothesis (Hall, 1975) has not received

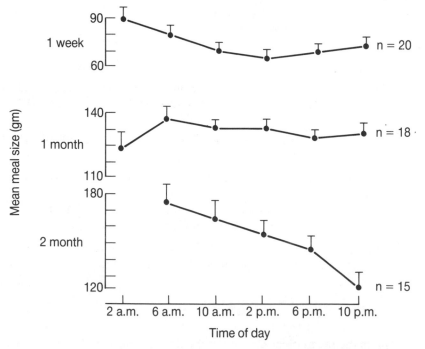

Fig 4.3   Mean meal size of breast feeds plotted at 4-hourly intervals over a 24-hour period

Table 4.2 Mothers' prior awareness of hunger variation (8 weeks postpartum)

	Male	Female
Yes	27	32
No	13	1

$\chi^2 = 8.32$ (1 d.f.) $p < 0.01$

any experimental support (Wooldridge, et al, 1980). Indeed, we have evidence from one infant, who was bottle fed after 10 weeks of age without any restriction on the availability of milk, that the same changes with age can appear with formula feeding and, therefore, cannot be due to changes in the nature of the milk itself (Wright, 1987a).

When the hunger ratings that the mothers gave at each meal were examined, it was found that, in the same way that the meal patterns alter from being equal across the day at 1 month old to a pronounced diurnal pattern at 8 weeks of age, the hunger ratings behave in identical fashion. It is also possible to look at how mothers answered the three questions in the survey before they began to keep these records, and to see whether there is any agreement between their answers and the actual feeding patterns of the infants. At 8 weeks of age there was an unexpected and very clear sex difference in the mothers' reports of hunger variation: if they had a female infant, all but one of the mothers stated that there was a particular time of day when they felt their baby was more hungry than at any other time (Table 4.2), but if the infant was male, approximately 30% of the mothers reported that they were unaware of any differences in hunger across the day, often saying that he was ravenous all the time or not especially interested in any feed. At this age no mother chose to respond in terms of the baby being *less* hungry at any particular time, and there was no indication of any sex difference in reporting awareness of less milk.

The next problem was to assess how correct these statements were by comparing the mothers' answers with the actual records of milk intake and hunger ratings for the six time periods. Using a simple scoring technique (Wright, 1986), it was found that only about 30% were correct on an intake measure, and just under 50% on the ratings and also for milk availability. Multiparous mothers were slightly more accurate than those with only one infant, but this was not statistically significant. However, the actual correlation between hunger ratings and intake was significant at $p<0.05$ level and beyond in about two-thirds of the sample, irrespective of sex, and bore no relation to the mothers' prior statements about hunger, etc.

The mothers have a wide range of behaviour and reasons that they say indicate hunger in their infants, and these can be roughly broken down into five categories:

1. *Avidity measures* – refers to the intensity of the sucking or the speed or duration of sucking: 'desperate, sucks everything', 'sucks rapidly, sucks slowly and rhythmically'.
2. *Distractability* – the baby is deemed to be more hungry because it is less

Table 4.3 Time of day when the baby was more hungry (at 2 months of age)

	Female	Male
Afternoon/late evening	18	9
First meal in morning	10	7

$\chi^2 = 4.19$ (1 d.f.) $p < 0.05$

distractable and more single minded about its feeding: 'gets on with it', 'sustained concentration', 'no rests for looking about'.
3. *Cries and screams* – 'cries and will not be distracted', 'screams until fed'.
4. *Very frequent feeding* – the baby is hungry because he or she demands the breast more frequently: 'wants lots of little feeds', 'has to be fed very often'.
5. *Cognitive reasoning* – the baby has gone a long time without food and, therefore, must be more hungry.

At this age the most frequently stated reason for female infants being viewed as hungry (11 out of 32 cases) was 'very frequent feeding', and for the male infants 8 out of 27 mothers opted for 'cries and screams'. If the time of day when the mothers report that their infants are most hungry is examined, it is normally early morning or late afternoon/early evening, and when only these two periods are considered (Table 4.3), the female infants are likely to be reported as being more hungry in the afternoon/evening than in the morning, whereas the ratio is roughly equal for males.

So, by 8 weeks of age females have developed a pronounced diurnal rhythm of meal size and are almost all reported as definitely having a particular time of day when they seem more hungry, the most common reason offered by their mothers for this being that they feed more frequently at this time, which is usually around late afternoon and early evening. In male infants, the same pattern appears somewhat later, and they appear to be more reluctant to drop feeds occurring between midnight and 4 a.m.

Because at 1 month of age, the mean meal size across the day is constant, it was expected that mothers would not report a high degree of variation in hunger, but in fact 77% of the mothers did report hunger varying across the day. The sample was smaller than for the 8-week-old babies, and this time the mothers reported greater awareness of change if the babies were male (Table 4.4). Yet despite this apparent reversal between the two ages, the 'correctness' of the mothers' judgments was much greater for females than for males (Wright, 1986).

The mothers of female infants do seem more in tune with their babies' expressed hunger behaviour than do the mothers of males. This might be due to misinterpreting high levels of activity and high arousal with hunger. In one direct study of Expressive behaviours associated with the period immediately before and after a meal, Korner (1973) found that in the first week of life girls were significantly more likely to engage in hand-to-mouth activity before meals than were boys. Perhaps this increased frequency of expressive behaviour associated with hunger is more appar-

Table 4.4 Baby's hunger variation across the day (at 4 weeks old)

	Yes	No
Male	14	0
Female	9	7

$\chi^2 = 5.73$ (1 d.f.) $p < 0.02$

ent to mothers of girls, leads to their increased awareness of hunger signals in general and explains the broad agreement between beliefs and measures of intake that we have described here.

CONCLUSIONS

A number of findings on how the feeding behaviour of infants appears to change with age have been summarised above. The most dramatic of these changes seem to occur between about 5 and 7 weeks of age, when the infants change from a fairly constant meal size whatever the time of day, to consuming large meals in the very early morning and then progressively smaller meals as the day progresses. It is this age that was identified at the beginning of the chapter as representing the critical transition point between unsuccessful and successful breast feeding. Very few mothers seem aware of these developmental changes and neither do the midwives and health visitors. As a likely accompaniment of the developmental shifts in meal pattern is increased fractiousness and frequent feeding in the late afternoon and early evening, mothers who know of these changes will be less likely to attribute difficulties to their own failure to produce a sufficient milk supply. A more accurate picture of what breast feeding entails should prevent unrealistic expectations, might well improve mothers' success as breast feeders and promote a more positive attitude towards their abilities as mothers. In the terms of the social psychology literature on attitude change, such a strategy could be seen as an attempt to 'inoculate' the mothers against the abandonment of their originally stated desire to breast feed in the face of the inevitable problems (Macguire, 1965). An attitude espoused in response to both negative and positive arguments and evidence (in this case, the wish to breast feed and the belief that it is 'best for baby') will be more resistant to change than one based on positive information alone. The central aim of any postnatal education programme should, therefore, be to prepare mothers to anticipate and be prepared to cope with the problems and realities of breast feeding, as well as reinforcing knowledge already acquired.

ACKNOWLEDGEMENT

The author would like to thank the Moray Fund, University of Edinburgh, for partial support of this work.

REFERENCES

Black, P.M., Faulkner, A.M. and Thomson, A.M. (1984) Antenatal classes: a selective review of the literature. *Nurse Education Today*, **3**: 130–133.

Crow, R.A. (1977) An ethological study of the development of infant feeding. *Journal of Advanced Nursing*, **2**: 99–109.

Crow, R.A. and Wright, P. (1976) The development of feeding behaviour in early infancy. *Nursing Mirror*, **142**: 57–59.

Department of Health and Social Security (1980) *Present Day Practice in Infant Feeding: 1980*, Report on Health and Social Subjects No. 20. London: HMSO.

Department of Health and Social Security (1989) *Present Day Practice in Infant Feeding: Third Report*, No. 32. London: HMSO.

Dunn, J. (1975) Consistency and change in styles of mothering. In: *Parent–Infant Interaction*, Ciba Symposium 33, pp. 155–170. Amsterdam: Elsevier.

Hall, B. (1975) Changing composition of human milk and early development of an appetite control. *The Lancet*, **i**: 779–781.

Korner, A.F. (1973) Sex differences in newborns with special reference to differences in the organisation of oral behaviour. *Journal of Child Psychology and Psychiatry*, **14**: 19–29.

Macguire, W.J. (1965) Inducing resistance to persuasion. In: *Advances in Experimental Social Psychology*, Berkowitz, L. (ed.). London: Academic Press.

McIntosh, J. (1985) Barriers to breastfeeding: choice of feeding method in a sample of working class primiparae. *Midwifery*, **1**: 213–224.

Martin, J. and Monk, J. (1982) *Infant Feeding 1980*. Office of Population Censuses and Surveys, Social Survey Division. London: HMSO.

Martin, J. and White, A. (1988) *Infant Feeding 1985*. Office of Population Censuses and Surveys, Social Survey Division. London: HMSO.

Newson, J. and Newson, E. (1963) *Patterns of Infant Care in an Urban Community*. London: Penguin.

Paul, A. and Whitehead, R. (1986) The weighting game. *Nursing Times, Community Outlook*, **July**: 11–17.

Richards, M.P.M. and Bernal, J. (1972) An observational study of mother–infant interaction. In: *Ethological Studies of Child Behaviour*, Blurton-Jones, N. (ed.). Cambridge: Cambridge University Press.

Sacks, S.H., Brada, M., Hill, A.M., Barton, P. and Harland, P.S.E.G. (1976) To breast feed or not to breast feed. *Practitioner*, **216**: 183–191.

West, C.P. (1980) Factors influencing the duration of breast feeding. *Journal of Biosocial Science*, **12**: 325–331.

Wooldridge, M.W., Baum, J.D. and Drewett, R.F. (1980) Does a change in the composition of human breast milk affect sucking patterns and milk intake? *The Lancet*, **ii**: 1292–1294.

Wright, P. (1981) Development of feeding behaviour in early infancy: implications for obesity. *Health Bulletin*, **39**: 197–206.

Wright, P. (1986) Do breast-feeding mothers know how hungry their babies are? *Midwifery*, **2**: 86–92.

Wright, P. (1987a) Hunger, satiety and feeding behaviour in early infancy. In: *Eating Habits*, Boakes, R.A., Barton, M. and Popplewell, R., pp. 75–106. Chichester: John Wiley and Sons.

Wright, P. (1987b) Editorial: Breast feeding behaviour and knowledge. *Journal of Reproductive and Infant Psychology*, **5**: 125–126,.

Wright, P. (1988) Learning experiences in feeding behaviour during infancy. *Journal of Psychosomatic Medicine*, **32**: 613–619.

Wright, P. and Crow, R.A. (1982) Nutrition and feeding. In: *Psychobiology of the Human Neonate*, Stratton, P. (ed.). Chichester: John Wiley and Sons.

Wright, P., Fawcett, J. and Crow, R.A. (1980) The development of differences in the feeding behaviour of bottle and breast-fed human infants. *Behavioural Processes*, **5**: 1–20.

5

POSTNATAL DEPRESSION: THE HEALTH VISITOR AS COUNSELLOR

Jenifer Holden

THE AIMS OF THE RESEARCH

The aims of the research focused on ways to help primary care workers to meet the needs of women with postnatal depression. The first aim was to develop a simple self-report scale that could be used to screen women for postnatal depression, and the second to determine whether or not a health visitor counselling intervention would be helpful to depressed mothers. The research was based in the University Department of Psychiatry in Edinburgh.

INTRODUCTION TO POSTNATAL DEPRESSION

In recent years there has been an encouraging upsurge of interest in postnatal depression. However, research interest is not necessarily reflected in improved patient care: three prospective studies in Edinburgh and London (Cox et al, 1982; Kumar and Robson, 1984; Watson et al, 1984) showed that although more than one in 10 women were found to have postnatal depression, few were identified or treated. The establishment of self-help groups (such as the Association for Postnatal Illness) shows the seriousness with which mothers themselves regard the condition and may indicate their lack of confidence in existing services.

As with any depression, the postnatal manifestation is characterised by loss of sleep, loss of concentration, loss of temper, loss of appetite and loss of the pleasure response, including that of love-making. However, it differs from depression occurring at other times of life in that its effects are experienced at a time when exceptional physical and emotional demands are being made on the mother.

When aked to describe her experience, one mother said:

'It was horrible. I didn't know what was wrong with me. It was like someone else living inside my body. The way you feel, it's as if you are going mad. I can now understand people who try to kill themselves. I couldn't be bothered with my husband and I had no time for the children; I never wanted to actually hurt them, but I did get very angry with them, which isn't like me at all.'

Postnatal depression is not only an unpleasant and disabling experience for the woman herself but can also have long-term effects on the family. Although postnatal depression only rarely leads to non-accidental injury and most depressed mothers manage to cope with routine tasks, they do not have the energy to play with their children or talk to them. Maternal depression can affect the baby's social and intellectual development and also that of other children in the family. It can also jeopardise the relationship between the parents. In contrast to the anticipated joys of parenthood, the father finds that his partner is irritable, withdrawn and unresponsive. While some fathers respond with support and help, others feel helpless and rejected and, finding it hard to accept their partner's apparent change of personality, may begin to avoid her company or even leave home.

There are many reasons why postnatal depression is not identified. The social isolation experienced by many mothers not only contributes to their depression but also enables it to pass unnoticed by those outside the family. Professionals may miss postnatal depression unless they are actively looking for its presence: midwives and doctors may concentrate on the mother's physical rather than emotional well-being, and health visitors may be preoccupied with the developmental progress of the baby. Hennessy (1985) found that health visitors had only recognised the condition in 27% of mothers she identified as depressed. Even if depressed women realise that help is available, they may be reluctant to confide, fearing the stigma associated with mental illness or imagining that they will be judged as inadequate. Media representations of happy motherhood make depression seem like a personal failure. One woman in our study said:

> 'I went down to my GP to ask for help; I said, "Right, I am going to tell him what is going on", but I got myself into that much of a state that I never said anything. I was getting cramp in my stomach at the time and I just told him about that. I just couldn't bring myself to tell him, I just couldn't.'

The implications of depression for the mother herself are sufficient for it to merit special attention. If we also take into consideration the long-term harmful effects that depression at this time may have on the family unit, it can be seen that the early diagnosis and active treatment of postnatal depression should be a matter of the highest priority. For these reasons the aim was to design a self-report scale to help professionals to identify mothers with postnatal depression.

DEVELOPMENT OF THE EDINBURGH POSTNATAL DEPRESSION SCALE (EPDS)

(See also Cox et al, 1987.)

Depression questionnaires that people can fill in themselves are widely used in clinical settings and in research. The aim was to develop a scale that would not only reliably identify postnatal depression but would also be short, simple and acceptable to non-depressed as well as depressed women.

Method

The pilot questionnaire consisted of 21 items, some new and others adapted from existing scales. After extensive testing at baby clinics the number of items was reduced to 10 simple statements relating to symptoms of depression. Each item has four possible responses, the mother being asked to underline the response that comes closest to how she has felt during the past week. The items are scored from 0 to 3 and are totalled to give an overall score.

Validation of the EPDS

The EPDS was completed in 84 postnatal women from the case loads of health visitors in Livingston and Edinburgh. The women were given a Standardised Psychiatric Interview (Goldberg et al, 1970) by the research psychiatrist, depression being classified according to Research Diagnostic Criteria (Spitzer et al, 1975).

Results

The EPDS reliably identified postnatal depression. Eighty-six per cent of depressed mothers scored over 12, 78% of non-depressed mothers scored 12 or below, and 73% of the mothers who scored more than 12 were depressed. Thus the sensitivity was 86%, the positive predictive value 73% and the specificity 78%. The scale proved to be simple to administer, to complete and to score and was acceptable to both the women and the health visitors.

Sensitivity to Change Over Time

It is important to know whether a self-report scale can be used on a subsequent occasion to elicit whether the individual is still depressed or whether she is getting better. Three months after the first interview the EPDS and the psychiatric interview were repeated with 31 women who had been identified as depressed. Comparing the mean EPDS scores at the first and second interview, those of the 15 mothers who were still depressed decreased from 16.5 to 15.4 (not significantly different), while those of the 16 mothers who had recovered dropped from 15.8 to 9.8 (t = 3.72, $p < 0.002$). This shows that the EPDS can be used to detect changes in the severity of depression over time.

Discussion

The EPDS is a simple and effective way of finding out whether or not women are suffering from postnatal depression. Use of the scale should always be combined with clinical judgment; a high score does not in itself constitute a diagnosis. The EPDS does, however, provide a useful introduction to a discussion of how the mother is feeling and can be used to identify women who need further assessment. The EPDS asks how the mother has felt during the previous week and may be repeated after 2 weeks. A score of 12 or over on two occasions almost certainly indicates a need for intervention. The sensitivity of the EPDS to changes in the severity of depression makes it a useful monitor for progress in treatment.

During the intervention study the self-report depression scale was incorporated into clinic routines by health visitors. It was well accepted by the women, many of whom reported having been relieved at being asked to complete it, feeling that this indicated an interest in them as individuals and gave them permission to speak about their feelings. One mother said:

> 'I filled it in automatically. It was good; I felt I'd told somebody, that someone knew how I felt. When my health visitor came and asked how I was, I told her I was fed up. I could tell her because I'd filled in the form. I'd felt bottled up like a schoolgirl – don't speak until you're spoken to.'

THE COUNSELLING STUDY

(See also Holden et al, 1989.)

Having found a way of detecting postnatal depression, ways to help depressed women were next considered. During the EPDS validation study, depressed women reported that they felt much better after having the opportunity to talk about their feelings in the psychiatric interview, and the literature supports the view that therapeutic listening can help depressed people. Brown and Harris (1978) pointed out the importance of having a confidant, and the lack of a confiding relationship has been shown to be associated with postnatal depression. We consulted community based psychologists and psychiatric nurses, who said that although counselling is certainly beneficial in postnatal depression, their services cannot meet the needs of the one in 10 mothers who become depressed. It has been suggested that as health visitors are already involved with mothers postnatally, they may be the people best placed to intervene in postnatal depression. The researchers, therefore, decided to find out whether or not health visitors could usefully offer counselling to mothers with postnatal depression.

Preparation for the Study

General practitioners and nursing managers were consulted, and 17 health visitors, working in two health centres in Livingston and three in Edinburgh, agreed to take on the key role of counsellors in the study. Some expressed concern as to the extra time that would be involved but it was estimated that each health visitor should be asked to counsel no more than three depressed mothers overall. The health visitors felt that their involvement would not only help their own understanding of postnatal depression but might also increase awareness of the condition among fellow professionals.

The health visitors also expressed interest in learning more about counselling. Ferguson (1988) found that health visitors regard much of their work as counselling. However, the majority of health visitors in this study expressed their need for additional training and this has also been mentioned by Burnard (1987). Health visitors in our study who had been trained for some years said that they had been given little information about counselling, while those who had trained more recently felt that they had learned an information-gathering rather than a non-directive counselling approach. Two health visitors had had additional counselling training and one planned to train as a psychosexual counsellor.

Instruction for Counselling

The main aim of the teaching sessions was to standardise the health visitors' approach to counselling. Notes on the Rogerian method of non-directive counselling (Holden, 1986) provided an introduction to the three instruction sessions, which consisted of discussion, role play and videos made with the help of the research psychiatrist. The principle underlying the non-directive approach is that sharing her feelings with an empathic and non-judgmental person helps the client to analyse her problems and find her own solutions. In this type of counselling the relationship between client and counsellor is more important than are specific techniques. Our aim was to encourage the health visitors to explore their own concerns about counselling and to build on their existing interpersonal skills, rather than to provide detailed instructions. Most importantly, we wanted the health visitors to encourage mothers to talk about how they were feeling and to listen constructively rather than making suggestions.

Design of the Counselling Study

Seven hundred and thirty-four women attending five health centres in Livingston and Edinburgh were asked by their health visitor to fill in an EPDS at the postnatal clinic approximately 6 weeks after delivery. Of these, 117 high-scoring women were then interviewed at home by the research psychiatrist approximately 13 weeks postnatally, using the same Standardised Psychiatric Interview. Fifty-five depressed mothers were allocated, using a system of random numbers, to the counselled group or the control group. General practitioners were informed of all depressed women but were not told to which group the women had been assigned. Health visitors were only told about women in the counselling group.

Women in the treatment group received up to eight sessions of non-directive counselling from their health visitor. The health visitor called weekly to allow the mother to talk for at least half an hour about how she was feeling, baby care being discussed at another time. It was stressed that privacy was important and that, if possible, the woman should ask someone to look after her baby and/or toddler(s) during this time.

The health visitors kept records of the counselling visits, and one of the researchers visited each health centre regularly to provide support. After the intervention (or an approximately equivalent time interval in the case of mothers in the control group) the mothers were reassessed by the research psychiatrist, who did not know to which group they had been allocated.

Description of the Sample

Of the 55 women taken into the study, 50 completed the trial, of whom 26 were in the counselled group and 24 in the control group. The women's mean age was 26 years (ranging from 16 to 40 years). Thirty-six had a normal spontaneous vertex delivery, 9 were delivered by caesarian section and 5 had a forceps delivery. One baby was born at home. According to their partner's occupation, 6 women were from social class II, 20 from social class III, and 24 from social classes IV and V.

Forty-seven women were married or living with a permanent partner and 4 were single. Twelve of the two-parent families and all the single women had no earned income. Parity and social factors were evenly distributed between the groups.

Results of the Counselling Study

The main finding from the study was that after a mean time interval of 13 weeks between the first and second diagnostic interview, two-thirds of the counselled women had recovered, compared to only one-third of the control group:

Counselled group (N = 26): 18 recovered and 8 remained depressed.
Control group (N = 24): 9 recovered and 15 remained depressed.

The superior rate of recovery for mothers in the counselling group was statistically significant ($\chi^2 = 5.06$, $p = 0.03$).

Discussion

Although confidence in the robustness of the findings should be tempered by the relatively small sample size, the superior recovery rate of counselled mothers indicates that health visitors can intervene effectively in the treatment of postnatal depression.

How Did the Mothers Respond?

Three months after the second psychiatric diagnosis had been made, tape-recorded interviews were held with all the women to discuss their participation in the study. At 15 interviews, the partner was also present. The women's comments indicated clearly the therapeutic role played by the health visitors.

One of the questions asked was: 'Did you get any help when you were depressed?' All 26 counselled women, but only 13 (54%) of controls, said that taking part in the study had been helpful. Twenty-four of the 26 counselled women (92%) said that talking to their health visitor had helped them most, and 3 even claimed that the health visitor had saved their marriage.

Twenty-two counselled women reported that participating in the study had changed their perception of the health visitor's job and of her approachability. Whereas previously they had considered that the health visitor came primarily to check on the baby's progress, they now realised that she was also there for them. One woman said:

'When my health visitor first came to the house, I thought she was a bit officious. She seemed so competent, so good at dealing with the baby. She kept telling me things to do with the baby, and I thought she meant I was doing it wrongly . . . Then when I was depressed, she came every week. I found her very easy to talk to and she didn't seem to be shocked by anything I said. It was such a relief to talk it out. Now I could talk to her about anything.'

How Did the Health Visitors Respond?

Most health visitors felt positively about their participation and reported feeling more confident in the role of counsellor than they did before. Many said they had found the non-directive approach useful in many areas of their work. However, in our short training we were only able to give an outline of actual techniques, and the health visitors were almost unanimous in their demand for more counselling input and for more information about postnatal depression during their training. One reported:

'Being in the study has made me even more acutely aware of the need for counselling training in the preparation of health visitors and in their future development in post. Our general practitioners would like us to be qualified counsellors. It is an unclaimed corner of the NHS market, which nurses should most appropriately claim as theirs.'

Conclusions

From this study it appears that health visitors who are given information about postnatal depression and basic instructions in non-directive counselling can have a considerable impact on the lives of mothers with postnatal depression. The use of the EPDS as a screen for postnatal depression was readily accepted by most mothers, and it could, without too much disruption (although with a good deal of organisation and determination) become part of the routine procedure of health visitors. However, the design of the study meant that the EPDS was scored by the researchers rather than by the health visitors themselves, and further study is needed to determine whether or not screening with the EPDS could become part of routine postnatal care.

In this study the majority of mothers saw the health visitor as being there mainly to make sure that the baby was progressing satisfactorily. Although many of the depressed mothers in the control group had a good relationship with their health visitor, most said they would be inhibited from telling her how they were feeling. It seems clear that most women need to be given explicit permission and a suitable opportunity before they are able to confide; even when offered counselling sessions some found it initially difficult to open up. However, once trust and acceptance were established, confiding their feelings not only made a significant difference in terms of reduction in clinical depression but also, in many cases, changed the women's perception of the role of the health visitor. Counselling was also described by many mothers as having had a beneficial effect on their relationship with their partner, and some said that it enabled them to talk to other people about their depression.

The study illuminated the need for more information about the realities of parenthood and the possibility and symptoms of postnatal depression to be given antenatally to parents. Four couples parted company during the research, and two of these were in the counselled group. This needs more study, possibly an intervention designed to include fathers, some of whom reported having felt discounted as no-one had asked how they were coping.

The study also revealed the need for back-up and support for health visitors offering counselling to depressed clients. Empathy involves participation in the distress of others and carers need help in coping with their own responses. Also, counselling is not the complete answer to postnatal depression: referral to psychiatric services should be readily available to women who need more help.

Overall, the results of this study have implications for the education of health visitors in the recognition of postnatal depression and the value of counselling. Mothers need to be given permission to talk about their feelings, but it is perhaps equally important that health professionals should be given permission as well as knowledge to enable them to listen effectively.

ACKNOWLEDGEMENTS

The research team, Professor J. Cox, Dr R. Sagovsky and Ms J. Holden, are indebted to the Scottish Home and Health Department, who funded the research, to the general practitioners and especially to the health visitors in Livingston and Edinburgh who collaborated so conscientously with us. Also grateful thanks go to Marjory Dodd and Richard Bambridge for their untiring support and to Ralph McGuire for his help with statistics.

REFERENCES

Brown, G.W. and Harris, T. (1978) *Social Origins of Depression*. London: Tavistock.
Burnard, P. (1987) The health visitor as counsellor: a framework for interpersonal skills. *Health Visitor*, **60**(8): 269.
Cox, J.L., Connor, Y. and Kendell, R.E. (1982) Prospective study of the psychiatric disorders of childbirth. *British Journal of Psychiatry*, **140**: 111–117.
Cox, J.L., Holden, J.M. and Sagovsky, R. (1987) Detection of postnatal depression: development of the 10-item Edinburgh Postnatal Depression Scale. *British Journal of Psychiatry*, **150**: 782–786.
Ferguson, A. (1986) Counselling: theoretical concepts and health visitors' perceptions. *Health Visitor*, **59**(4): 110–112.
Goldberg, D.P., Cooper, B., Eastwood, M.R., Kedward, H.B. and Shepherd, M.A. (1970) A standardised psychiatric interview for use in community surveys. *British Journal of Preventive and Social Medicine*, **24**: 18–23.
Hennessy, D.A. (1985) Should health visitors also care for mothers? In: *Proceedings of the RCN Research Society Annual Conference*, University of Nottingham, Hawthorne, P.J. (ed.). London: RCN.
Holden, J.M. (1986) Counselling notes for health visitors. In: *Postnatal Depression – A Guide for Health Professionals*, Cox, J.L., pp. 53–57. Edinburgh: Churchill Livingstone.
Holden, J.M., Sagovsky, R.S. and Cox, J.L. (1989) Counselling in a general practice setting: a controlled trial of health visitor intervention in postnatal depression. *British Medical Journal*, **298**: 233–236.
Kumar, R. and Robson, K.M. (1984) A prospective study of emotional disorders in childbearing women. *British Journal of Psychiatry*, **144**: 35–47.
Spitzer, R., Endicott, J. and Robins, E. (1975) *Research Diagnostic Criteria Instrument No. 58.* New York: New York Psychiatric Institute.
Watson, J.P., Elliot, S.A., Rugg, A.J. and Brough, D.I. (1984) Psychiatric disorder in pregnancy and the first postnatal year. *British Journal of Psychiatry*, **144**: 453–462.

6

THE MIDWIFERY PROCESS

Ros Bryar

BACKGROUND TO THE STUDY

During the 1970s, senior midwives at the study hospital became increasingly concerned about the practice of midwifery, and it is evident that this concern, which some felt as a crisis in midwifery, has continued into the mid-1980s (Association of Radical Midwives, 1986). The main issues of concern were: the erosion or invasion of the role of the midwife, particularly in care of the woman experiencing an uncomplicated pregnancy (Robinson et al, 1983); consumer dissatisfaction with the lack of attention to their individual needs (National Childbirth Trust, 1981); fragmentation of care between the hospital and community and between different staff within the hospital, contributing to the lack of identification of individual needs (Flint, 1979; Newton et al, 1979); the levels of infant mortality and morbidity (Department of Health and Social Security, 1976); and the problems of defining the staffing levels necessary to provide a high standard of care (Moores, 1980).

Similar issues had concerned nurses and had led to the development of the nursing process and patient allocation (de la Cuesta, 1979; Kratz, 1979). The literature on the use of the nursing process in midwifery was sparse (Methven, 1982). Senior midwives in the study hospital decided (initially in collaboration with a team of nurse researchers) to undertake a study of the introduction and use of the nursing process and 'patient' allocation. A research midwife was appointed for the 3-year project. During the first 2½ years of the project, the nursing process and 'patient' allocation were introduced into the work of midwifery and nursing staff within the hospital and community midwifery service. A cross-sectional study was then undertaken to assess the effects of the changes made.

Changes in Organisations

This study is concerned with the introduction of change to an organisation: a midwifery unit. Organisations have been analysed as bureaucracies, systems and professional organisations (Silverman, 1972). Silverman has proposed an action analysis of organisations. In this model, the action of the organisation, or members within the organisation, is considered to be dependent on the interaction between the changing stock of knowledge outside the organisation, the organisational role system and the individual's attachments and definitions of the situation, based on her wider experiences and experiences within the organisation. As illustrated in

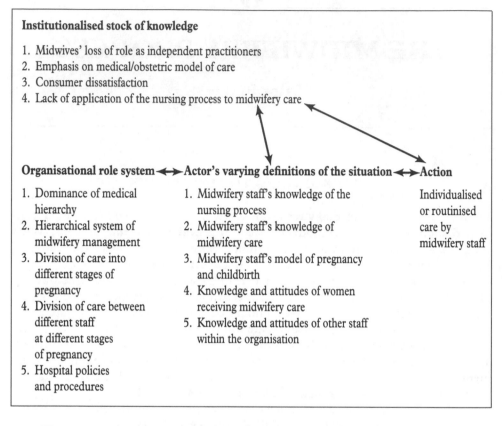

Institutionalised stock of knowledge

1. Midwives' loss of role as independent practitioners
2. Emphasis on medical/obstetric model of care
3. Consumer dissatisfaction
4. Lack of application of the nursing process to midwifery care

Organisational role system ⟷ Actor's varying definitions of the situation ⟷ Action

Organisational role system	Actor's varying definitions of the situation	Action
1. Dominance of medical hierarchy	1. Midwifery staff's knowledge of the nursing process	Individualised or routinised care by midwifery staff
2. Hierarchical system of midwifery management	2. Midwifery staff's knowledge of midwifery care	
3. Division of care into different stages of pregnancy	3. Midwifery staff's model of pregnancy and childbirth	
4. Division of care between different staff at different stages of pregnancy	4. Knowledge and attitudes of women receiving midwifery care	
5. Hospital policies and procedures	5. Knowledge and attitudes of other staff within the organisation	

Fig. 6.1   Factors affecting an organisation in its provision of individualised care

Figure 6.1, the changes introduced in the study resulted from changes in the wider body of knowledge outside the organisation. The changes were introduced to the work of individuals in one occupational group in the organisation. The model suggests that the changes may have different meanings and consequences for those individuals, depending on their previous experiences. Individuals occupying different role positions within the organisation will also be affected by the changes. The type of care provided will be dependent on the interaction of these different factors.

The Study Hospital and Community

The study hospital was a city maternity unit with a long midwifery and obstetric tradition and a reputation for providing high technology obstetric care. It was a 161-bedded unit divided into the wards and departments traditional to maternity units. The hospital-based community midwives provided midwifery care in an adjacent inner city health district. Midwifery care was provided by midwives and nurses, including enrolled nurses, nursery nurses, student midwives, student nurses, registered nurses undertaking the obstetric nursing course and auxiliaries. These staff are referred to in the following discussion as the midwifery staff.

Care was organised on task-orientated lines. Different teams of midwifery staff undertook care of the child-bearing woman in the antenatal clinic, antenatal ward, labour ward, postnatal wards and community. Within these teams, care was further divided. For example, on her first visit to the antenatal clinic, a woman was seen by a minimum of six midwifery staff, who undertook various tasks.

The Introduction of Change

Change was introduced by means of a programme of in-service education in which the nursing process and various forms of patient allocation were discussed. During early sessions, a midwifery assessment and care plan were devised and tested by staff. In the first year of the study, pilot projects of various assessment formats, care plans and methods of staff–woman allocation were held in different areas of the hospital and community. By the end of the first year, a midwifery assessment form containing information from the first antenatal visit to discharge from care postnatally by the community midwives had been finalised and was used in the care of all women from the beginning of the second year of the project. The care plan format was altered several times until the middle of the second year of the project, from which time a care plan covering care from the first antenatal visit to postnatal discharge was used.

In the antenatal clinic, each woman was allocated to a particular midwife for the whole of her antenatal care. On the antenatal and postnatal wards, women were allocated on a day-to-day basis to members of staff who were responsible for, as far as possible, the care of the same women each day. In the community, pairs of midwives worked together in attachment to particular general practices and covering particular geographical areas.

To support these changes, meetings were held each month, at which midwifery staff and social workers discussed the progress of the project. A co-ordinating group of nursing officers and tutorial staff was also established in the second year of the project (Adams et al, 1981; Bryar and Strong, 1983).

In the third year of the project a cross-sectional study was undertaken with the following aims:

1. To assess the extent to which a systematic approach to midwifery care, i.e. the nursing process approach with patient allocation, had been introduced into care provided by midwifery/nursing staff at the research hospital.
2. To examine the views of midwifery staff, other staff and clients about this approach.

The questions examined in this study were:

1. What was the knowledge of, the attitudes towards and the use of the nursing process and patient allocation by midwifery staff?
2. What was the knowledge of and attitudes towards the nursing process and patient allocation of other staff?

3. To what extent was care individualised to the needs of the individual woman and family?
4. To what extent did the woman and her family participate in the woman's own care?
5. What factors appear to affect the introduction and use of an individualised approach to midwifery care?

In the following description, information will be presented relating mainly to question 3 above.

METHODS USED IN CROSS-SECTIONAL STUDY

Midwifery care is a complex activity and it was, therefore, decided to adopt the approach of naturalistic inquiry (Denzin, 1978) to collect data. Naturalistic inquiry necessitates the participation of the researcher in the research setting, with the aim of identifying concerns of individuals within that setting. Data are collected by various methods, e.g. participant observation and surveys, which allow the comparison of data. In this way methodological triangulation is achieved and the weaknesses of one method of data collection are compensated for by the strengths of an additional method used (Denzin, 1970).

Non-participant Observation

Non-participant observation was the main method used during the cross-sectional study (Stacey, 1969). The main aim of this observation was to obtain information about the use of the nursing process in midwifery care. At earlier stages in the project it had been observed that written records and reports of care differed from observed care. It was, therefore, considered important to observe midwifery practice directly. A problem of this method is that the observer may influence the activity being observed (Lofland, 1971). In the present study, the research midwife had been in the hospital for over 2 years and it is considered that her presence did not affect the activities observed.

Another problem may be the misinterpretation by the researcher of certain activities. The nursing/midwifery background of the researcher probably reduced this effect. It was also reduced by staff volunteering information about their activities after the period of observation.

Questionnaire

A questionnaire was designed to provide information on the midwifery staff's knowledge of and views about the nursing process and patient allocation. The questionnaire was divided into three sections covering general background information about the individual, the midwifery process and patient allocation. It was decided to use a questionnaire rather than interview staff in order to obtain the views of a larger number of staff than would have been possible if interviews had been undertaken.

Interviews

Focused interviews were held with a sample of women attending the hospital (case study women), nursing officers and non-midwifery staff. In the focused interview a fixed list of questions is asked but the questions may be rephrased and asked in an order appropriate to the interview (Denzin, 1970). This method allows more flexibility than does the structured interview but ensures that information is collected in relation to each question for every respondent.

The interviews with the case study women aimed to discover:

1. to what extent the woman had experienced continuity of care;
2. what problems she had experienced during her pregnancy and to what extent she felt that these problems had been recognised by midwifery staff;
3. what help (if any) she had received with these problems from midwifery staff.

The interviews with the nursing officers and non-midwifery staff aimed to provide information about their knowledge of the nursing process and patient allocation and their views on these methods.

Content Analysis of Midwifery Process Records

Use of the nursing process in practice may be demonstrated in the direct observation of care but should also be demonstrated in the midwifery records of that care. For this reason the midwifery process records of the case study women were analysed to identify:

1. the extent to which the midwifery assessment was complete;
2. the extent to which problems and/or needs were identified on the midwifery assessment and care plans;
3. the number and content of problems;
4. the number and content of aims;
5. the number and content of plan statements;
6. the number and content of implementation (action) statements;
7. the number and content of continuing assessment statements and their relationship to problem statements;
8. the number and content of evaluation statements.

The records were analysed using a format devised for the study. Although content analysis may appear to be a relatively straightforward means of evaluating care or the use of the nursing process, in practice it presents many difficulties (Ashworth, 1982; O'Neill, 1984). Data from content analysis should also be compared with data from other sources before conclusions are drawn (Holsti, 1968; Carey, 1972).

These four methods of data collection were used to provide information from a number of different perspectives on the use of the nursing process by the midwifery staff at the study hospital.

SAMPLE SIZES AND CHARACTERISTICS

Data were collected from different samples depending on the method of data collection. Convenience sampling was used in drawing all the samples. In convenience sampling subjects are selected because they happen to be present in the study site at the time of sampling (Abdellah and Levine, 1979). Convenience sampling was used because the study was concerned with examining the process and effects of change (the introduction of the nursing process) in a particular site rather than with seeking information generalisable to a wider population.

Non-participant Observation

Non-participant observation was carried out in the six areas of the hospital involved in the project: the antenatal clinic, antenatal ward, labour ward and three postnatal wards (both day and night) and the community. Length of observation in each area varied between 3 nights and 2 weeks, giving a total of 262 hours. Observation took place on early and late shifts and night duty. Staff to be observed were chosen to provide a representative picture of those working in each area. In total, 47 staff were observed for complete shifts or parts of shifts (Table 6.1).

Table 6.1   Occupations of staff observed in the study

Occupation	Number
Midwifery sisters	14
Staff midwives	11
Enrolled nurses	2
Nursery nurses	3
Student midwives	7
Obstetric nurse students	6
Auxiliaries	4
Total	47

The Questionnaire

The questionnaire was distributed to all midwifery staff, except auxiliaries, working in each of the areas in which observation took place. One hundred and thirty-three questionnaires were distributed to ward and community staff and 10 questionnaires (which were modified) to nursing officers and tutorial staff.

Unfortunately, only 43 (30%) of the questionnaires were completed (36 from ward staff and 7 from the nursing officers). It is not possible to state in what ways (if any) those staff who returned the questionnaire differed from the total sample. Twenty-five midwives completed the questionnaire or its modified form. At least one midwife responded from each area (Table 6.2). Twenty-four of the midwives held nursing qualifications in addition to a midwifery qualification, and 15 had additional midwifery or nursing qualifications. Only one enrolled nurse returned the questionnaire. All the student midwives were qualified nurses, as were all but two of the obstetric nurses.

Table 6.2   The characteristics of staff who returned the questionnaire

Occupation	Number	Age range	Time at study hospital
Midwives – full time	23 ⎫	24–59 years	6 months – 14 years
Midwives – part time	2 ⎭		
Enrolled nurses	1	–	–
Nursery nurses	5	19–26 years	3–21 months
Student midwives	7 ⎫	21–25 years	1–9 months
Obstetric nurses	5 ⎭		

Interviews

Interviews were held with all the nursing officers and tutorial staff in the hospital. Their ages ranged from 30 to 45 years and they had been at the hospital for between 1 and 14 years. Six had qualifications in addition to basic nursing and midwifery qualifications. The sample of non-midwifery staff interviewed is shown in Table 6.3.

The sample of 21 case study women was drawn from women in the six areas of observation (excluding the labour ward) who met the following criteria: were on the ward or under the care of the community midwives for most or all of the period of

Table 6.3   Non-midwifery staff interviewed

Occupation	Number
Ward clerks	4
Paediatric house officers	2
Obstetric house officers	3
Social workers	3
Physiotherapists	3
Total	15

observation; were women whose care could be observed (i.e. they or their baby was not seriously ill); spoke English; and agreed to be interviewed. These women were identified on the first day of observation in an area and were approached to be interviewed on the last day of the observation period.

In the antenatal clinic, women attending for examination towards the end of pregnancy were approached. No woman approached refused to be interviewed. A convenience sample of women was used as the population of women attending the

Table 6.4   The characteristics of the 21 case study women

Ages	16–40 years (median 30 years)
Multigravidae	13
Primigravidae	8
Stable relationships	19
Planned home confinement	1
Type of delivery	
LSCS	7
Forceps	4
Breech	1

hospital was so large that a completely separate study would have been required to gather data from a profitability sample (Table 6.4). Content analysis of the midwifery process records of the case study women was undertaken.

DATA COLLECTION

The research proposal was approved by the ethical committee of the study hospital. Data were collected between April and August 1982 by one research midwife using the various methods described above. During observation consent for observation to take place was obtained verbally from staff and women who were directly observed. An explanation of the project was given to these people. When observation was taking place in a ward women not being directly observed were given information about the project if they requested it. When interviews were undertaken verbal consent was again obtained for note-taking and women were asked if they had any objections to their records being examined. Staff who completed the questionnaires were assured that their replies would be treated in confidence.

Non-participant Observation

Data were collected by accompanying midwifery staff during a period of duty. Observations were recorded in a diary format in a notebook at the time or as soon after the event as possible. A record was made of care given by midwifery and other staff, ward organisation, ward reports and comments by staff and women relating to care and different approaches to care. Particular note was made of the care of the case study women. This open, non-participant observation was focused on midwifery care and the use of the nursing process and patient allocation in that care.

Questionnaire

The questionnaire was distributed to midwifery staff on the last day of the period of observation in each area and to nursing officers at their interview. Only 30% of the questionnaires were returned by the end of August. Several reasons may explain this poor response rate. The questionnaire took more than 1½ hours to complete and some staff (in comparison with students with whom the questionnaire was piloted) found some terms in the questionnaire difficult to understand. In addition, some staff commented that they considered they had given their opinions on the issues covered in the questionnaire during the period of observation. It is suggested that interviews with staff would be the method of choice were the study to be repeated.

Interviews

Interviews with the non-midwifery staff and nursing officers were held at the end of the period of data collection. The interviews were held in private at a time convenient to these staff. Notes were recorded of replies to questions during the interview. Interviews with the case study women were held at the end of the period of observation in an area. The interviews were held in the ward area or teaching room. In the antenatal clinic women were interviewed as they waited to be examined. Five women were interviewed at home following discharge from the care of the community midwives. During these interviews other people were frequently present, but their presence did not appear to affect the conduct of any interview. Answers to questions on the interview schedule were recorded in a notebook and, following the interview, reorganised to the order of the interview schedule. The interviews lasted between 25 minutes and 1 hour 25 minutes.

Records

Following their discharge from the hospital or from care of the community midwives, the midwifery process records of the case study women were extracted from their obstetric notes and photocopied. These 21 sets of midwifery assessments and care plans formed the data for the content analysis.

ANALYSIS AND RESULTS

The use of several methods of analysis generated a considerable number of data, which were analysed manually.

Observational Data

Observational notes were written up each day and, as this was done, initial analysis was begun with the recording of analytical comments when these were suggested by the data (Lofland, 1971). Later observation was used to test these ideas in practice. Full analysis was not undertaken until some time later.

The observational data were then examined in relation to a set of predetermined topics related to aspects of the nursing process, for example the participation of the women in problem/need identification. Other topics arose from the data, for example the effects of hospital policies on care (Dingwall, 1976). The data were then re-examined in relation to these new topics. Using the cut-and-stick method, the notes were reorganised under these topic headings. Each topic was then examined in relation to data obtained using the other methods.

Questionnaires

The questionnaires were analysed manually. Comments recorded in response to the open questions were categorised in relation to categories developed from the review of the literature. Simple statistics were calculated, which need to be examined with care considering the small number of responses to the questionnaires.

Interviews

The interviews with the three samples were analysed separately. The responses to the questions were categorised according to repeated themes and in relation to the literature.

Content Analysis

Both the midwifery assessment and care plans were analysed. The 132-item assessment was examined for completeness and also in relation to the identification of problems on the assessment. Each statement on the care plans was isolated and categorised according to the analysis framework. There was a total of 3344 statements on the care plans. The statements were first categorised in relation to a stage of the nursing process, e.g. problem, plan or action statement. Each statement was then further categorised; for example, problem statements were recorded as antenatal or postnatal problems, actual or possible problems, whether they were stated in vague terms, in some detail or individualised to a particular woman, and whether they were stated in terms that described the problem in medical or midwifery terms or in relation to the woman's or baby's problem.

At each stage of the data analysis, the data collected using one method were compared with data collected using an alternative method and with the literature. All analysis was undertaken by one person rather than several coders, which may influence the validity of the findings. Evidence, however, from the literature, for example of similar categories used for the analysis of records (O'Neill, 1984), suggests that the effects of bias may have been minimised by the use of different methods of data collection.

To what extent was care individualised to the needs of the individual woman and family?

Observation

On a minority of occasions during the period of observation individualised care planning and implementation of care was observed; for example, Student midwife F spent a considerable amount of time with Mrs 20 discussing the reasons for her admission to the antenatal ward, her home circumstances, etc. and discovered she had not attended any parentcraft classes. The student reported this at the ward report and later in the day took Mrs 20 to the class that she had expressed an interest in attending. At ward reports and while care was being given, alternative plans of care were discussed, e.g. care for cracked nipples.

In all areas, standardised care was observed. In some cases this care was determined by hospital policies, for example that babies should not be bathed until the fourth day:

> 'Mrs Y asked the nursery nurse if her baby's hair could be washed. The nursery nurse replied that she would do it in the afternoon. Mrs Y asked if the baby could have a bath. The nursery nurse replied that this was not done usually until the fourth day, but that she could give the hair a wash.' (Observation notes, postnatal ward)

Routine care was indicated by: written instructions about the frequency of observations; teaching of students, for example 'If bowels are not opened by the third day, then the women have suppositories' (staff midwife Z, observation notes, postnatal ward); and the giving of standardised information, often before an individual assessment had been made, for example:

'*Staff Midwive M*:   Are you taking iron?
Mrs. E: No.
Staff Midwife M: Probably a bit early yet; wait until your blood results are back before you start. If you are eating a good diet, you should be OK. Need lots of vegetables, you can't eat liver every day! But red meat is good. You're not a vegetarian, are you?
Mrs. E: No.'
(Observation notes, antenatal clinic)

Three other factors appeared to affect the care given: the structure of the ward or clinic day, the activities of other staff and the experience of those giving 'midwifery care'. For example, on the postnatal wards, all observations on the women and babies were completed by lunch time, which necessitated the postponement of bathing the babies until the afternoon. The individual needs of the women and babies, however, often thwarted this structure, as a student reported to a nursery nurse:

'all the babies for baths were sleeping and the woman with whom the student was going to do the demonstration was feeding and said she would like to watch today and do a bath tomorrow'. (Observation notes, postnatal ward)

The activities of other staff, for example obstetricians in the antenatal clinic, paediatricians and physiotherapists, appeared to take precedence over the care provided by midwifery staff. For example,

'Obstetric nurse K in room doing postnatal observations. Physiotherapist A said into room that she would take a class now unless obstetric nurse K was very busy. Obstetric nurse K made no comment but took the thermometer out of Mrs F's mouth and said to her that she would come back later.' (Observation notes, postnatal ward)

Many of the staff giving 'midwifery care' were students as well as nursery nurses, enrolled nurses and auxiliaries. It was observed that, particularly in the case of the students, lack of knowledge inhibited problem identification and care planning and this was expressed on several occasions by the students. For example, following a ward teaching session about signs of breast inflammation, a student commented in response to the staff midwife's suggestion that she now knew all about it, 'Yes, about as much as they [the women] do!'

Questionnaires

For the 43 staff who completed the questionnaire, it was found that their previous knowledge of and use of the nursing process was related to their age and qualifications. Thirteen of the 25 midwives, the five nursery nurses and the enrolled nurse had had no experience of the nursing process prior to the project. In contrast, only one of the 12 students had no previous knowledge of the nursing process.

From their replies to the questionnaire it appeared that the staff viewed the nursing process as a tool to help in the individualisation of care, although they identified problems with its use. Question 9 asked, 'How would you define the nursing process?' Twenty of the 43 descriptions defined the nursing process in terms of the identification of the total or individual needs of women, for example:

> 'The nursing process is a patient-centred method of identifying the particular needs of a particular person and of deciding the most effective way of meeting those needs, followed by an evaluation of the measures adopted in relation to the patient.' (Staff midwife H)

Similarly, in their descriptions of assessment, the majority referred to it as a process of gathering information about an individual, 'looking at each patient's individual history and isolating his or her problems' (Sister L).

Twenty-nine of the 36 ward staff responded positively to a question about the benefits of the nursing process. For example, use of the nursing process, by providing more information about each woman, allowed for easier care planning and increased the staff's knowledge of the women:

> 'It has made us think more of the woman as a person in a family unit by gleaning information about the psychosocial situation.' (Sister C)

Of the 36 staff, 32 considered the nursing process to be of benefit to the women. Twenty-seven, however, felt the benefit was indirect – that the nursing process helped the staff to know the women, which benefited the women.

Problems with the use of the nursing process were identified by 18 staff. These problems related to: the staff's lack of knowledge of the nursing process; organisational factors, including staffing levels and the rapid change of staff, appointment times in the antenatal clinic, etc.; and the fragmentation of care of the child-bearing woman:

> 'it is generally more difficult to introduce to a midwifery unit than a nursing one, perhaps due to the quick turnover of patients . . . It may be that we identify potential problems knowing that the care to prevent them will never be implemented due to early transfer home.' (Miss I)

Interviews

During the interviews the women were not asked directly about the individualisation of care but their comments in reply to some questions suggested they had experienced certain problems. Mrs 2, for example, commented on the procedure for bathing babies, which had changed since her previous delivery:

> 'Mrs 2 said that she had been shown how to bath the baby by the nursery nurse. The procedure had changed from last time when they used to use Infracare – now use soap, possibly to save money? The nursery nurse told her they had gone back to the old-fashioned methods. She found it difficult to soap the baby and put her in the water as she was very slippery. Does it her own way now at home by soaping the baby in the bath after putting her in.' (Interview notes)

Mrs 4 felt that staff on the postnatal ward only came to her when they had a task to perform. This contrasted with her experience on the antenatal ward where staff had spent a considerable amount of time with her.

There was evidence that problems were not identified or, if they were identified, no record was made of the problem for long-term care. For example, Mrs 8, a primigravida aged 27 years, at term, identified seven problems during the interview. During her examination in the antenatal clinic three of these were identified, adding to four other problems. The midwife spent some time discussing Mrs 8's problems but none of the problems or care implemented was recorded in the midwifery records. Similarly, in the case of Mrs 20 referred to above, no record was made in the midwifery records of her lack of knowledge of parentcraft, the care implemented to change this situation and her evaluation of the class, which she described during the interview as 'boring'.

Content Analysis

The midwifery assessment and care plan provide a written record of the care given and the individuality of that care. To provide individualised care a full assessment of each woman should be made. It was found that, on the 132-item midwifery assessment, only 19 items were completed for all the applicable women in the sample of 21. Thirteen items were completed for five or fewer of the 21 women to whom they were applicable. These included information on antenatal classes for five women and breast examination for two. In contrast, medical and obstetric history details and details of labour and delivery were the sections completed in most detail.

The midwifery assessments were examined by the research midwife and 142 problems were identified from the information on the assessments. Of these, 81 were categorised as actual problems, for example 'Worried for baby's health', and 61 as possible problems, for example 'Depression postnatally (previous pregnancy)'. Thirty-eight (27%) of these problems were recorded on the care plans.

When the care plans were examined, 230 problems were identified, of which 170 were recorded in the problem/need section of the care plan and 60 elsewhere. The following description refers to those in the problem/need section as they were the problems specifically identified by staff. Eighty-seven per cent of these problems were classified as physical, 12% as referring to emotional, social or educational needs and one problem referred to a problem relating to the family. For example:

'Cracked nipple' (*physical*)
'Looks tired, says she hasn't time for anything' (*emotional*)

Sixty-one per cent of the problems were written in vague terms, 27% contained more detail and only 12% were written in terms that individualised the problem to a particular woman. For example:

'Anxiety' (*vague*)
'Sore right nipple' (*more detail*)
'Pyrexia persists: 14.00, 37.5°C' (*individualised*)

When classified according to frame of reference, 34% were categorised as being written in terms of the woman's frame of reference, 36% in terms of a medical framework and 29% in terms of a midwifery framework, for example:

'Feeling tired' (*woman's framework*)
'Pre-eclamptic toxaemia' (*medical framework*)
'Postop immobilisation' (*midwifery framework*)

The lack of individuality and detail in the problem statements was reflected in the remainder of the statements on the care plans. For example, of the 58 aims recorded on the care plans, only 15 (26%) were classified as containing some detail of what outcome of care was expected. The remaining 43 (74%) were classified as being written in vague terms, and none was classified as being a measurable aim individualised to a particular woman or baby.

DISCUSSION

A description has been given of the introduction of the nursing process into the care provided by midwifery staff. Data presented from the assessment of the introduction of this change focused on the individualisation of care. The nursing process literature (for example, de la Cuesta, 1979) emphasises the individualisation of care as a major aspect of the nursing process. Evidence from consumers also suggests that they seek individualised care (National Childbirth Trust, 1981). Responses by midwifery staff showed that they valued individualised care and saw the nursing process as a tool to achieve such care.

The majority of the evidence from the non-participant observation undertaken suggested that care was routinised, and various factors restricting care were identified, including hospital policies, the structure of the ward day and the knowledge of those giving care. The care plans showed that there was a lack of identification of individual problems. Those problems that were identified were largely physical, as Laryea (1980) found in her study. The combination of observation and content analysis showed that there was a wide disparity between the large number of problems and care provided in practice and the lack of recording of problems and plans. Evidence from the interviews also suggested that care was not individualised. It is suggested that the use of different methods of data collection helped to provide a more complete picture of the use of the nursing process, evidence collected using one method being supported by evidence collected by a different method.

At the time of the cross-sectional study, the data collected showed that care provided by midwifery staff was routinised, orientated towards physical needs and unresponsive to individual needs. Care was fragmented between different teams of midwifery staff in different departments and within each department was fragmented between staff of different grades and experience. The nursing process, although understood to a considerable extent by the sample of staff, had not been fully implemented at the hospital. The midwifery staff were constrained in their ability to provide individualised care. The action framework (see Figure 6.1) demonstrates some of the intra- and extra-organisational constraints on change. The introduction of change via an educational programme, as in the present study, has been criticised (Hunt, 1982; Milne, 1985). Consideration of the intra- and extra-organisational factors affecting midwifery care, both prior to and during the process of change, may contribute to greater changes in the long term. The introduction of the nursing process is a gradual process. Since the end of the project, staff at the study hospital have continued the process of change and the reassessment of the cumulative changes made.

ACKNOWLEDGEMENTS

Thanks are extended to the administrators of the endowment funds at the study hospital who funded the 3-year study and to the Edwina Mountbatten Trust, which awarded a bursary that allowed time for data analysis. Miss Grace Owen and Miss Pat Ashworth provided invaluable supervision for the second year of the project. Particular thanks are extended to the staff at the study hospital who put so much into the project and who are continuing the process of change begun in this project.

REFERENCES

Abdellah, F.G. and Levine, E. (1979) *Better Patient Care through Nursing Research*, 2nd edn. New York: Macmillan.

Adams, M., Armstrong-Esther, C., Bryar, R., Duberley, J., Strong, G. and Ward, E. (1981) The nursing process in midwifery: trial run. *Nursing Mirror*, **153**(15): 32–35.

Ashworth, P. (1982) *Change from What? A Baseline Descriptive Study of Clinical Areas Involved with the UK (Manchester) Collaborating Centre in Research Associated with the WHO Medium Term Programme in Nursing/Midwifery in Europe*. Unpublished report. Copenhagen: WHO Regional Office.

Association of Radical Midwives (1986) *The Vision: Draft Proposal for the Future of the Maternity Services*, 3rd edn. London: Association of Radical Midwives.

Bryar, R. and Strong, G. (1983) Trial run – continued. *Nursing Mirror*, **157**(15): 45–48.

Carney, T.F. (1972) *Content Analysis. A Technique for Systematic Inference from Communications*. London: Batsford.

Cuesta, de la, C. (1979) *Nursing Process: From Theory to Implementation*. Unpublished MSc thesis, University of London.

Denzin, N.K. (1970) *The Research Act. A Theoretical Introduction to Research Methods*. Chicago: Aldine.

Denzin, N.K. (1978) *Sociological Methods. A Source Book*, 2nd edn. New York: McGraw-Hill.

Department of Health and Social Security (1976) *Prevention and Health. Everybody's Business*. London: HMSO.

Dingwall, R. (1976) The social organisation of health visitor training, 4: Method in nursing research. *Nursing Times*, Occasional Paper **72**(10): 37–40.

Flint, C. (1979) A team of midwives: a continuing labour of love. *Nursing Mirror*, **149**(2): 16–18.

Holsti, O.R. (1968) Content analysis. In: *The Handbook of Social Psychology*, Vol. 2, *Research Methods*, 2nd edn., Gardner, L. and Elliot, A. (eds.), Chapter 16. Reading, Massachusetts: Addison Wesley.

Hunt, M. (1982) An action research approach to promoting planned discharge of the elderly from acute wards to the community. In: *Proceedings of the RCN Research Society XIII Annual Conference, University of Durham*, Chapter 18. London: RCN.

Kratz, C.R. (ed.) (1979) *The Nursing Process*. London: Baillière Tindall.

Laryea, M.G.G. (1980) *The Midwives' Role in the Postnatal Care of Primiparae and their Infants in the First 28 Days following Childbirth*. Unpublished MPhil thesis, Newcastle-on-Tyne Polytechnic.

Lofland, J. (1971) *Analyzing Social Settings*. Belmont, California: Wadsworth.

Methven, R.C. (1982) *An Examination of the Content and Process of the Antenatal Booking Interview (Recording an Obstetric History or Relating with a Mother-to-be?)*. Unpublished MSc Thesis, University of Manchester.

Milne, D. (1985) 'The more things change the more they stay the same': factors affecting the implementation of the nursing process. *Journal of Advanced Nursing*, **10**(1): 39–45.

Moores, B. (1980) Towards rational midwifery service planning. *Journal of Advanced Nursing*, 5(3): 301–311.

National Childbirth Trust (1981) *Change in Antenatal Care*. London: NCT.

Newton, R.W., Webster, P., Binn, P., Maskrey, N. and Phillips, A. (1979) Psychosocial stress in pregnancy and its relation to the onset of premature labour. *British Medical Journal*, 2: 411–413.

O'Neill, J. (1984) *The Use of Nursing Records in the Evaluation of Nursing Care*. Unpublished MSc thesis, University of Manchester.

Robinson, S., Golden, J. and Bradley, S. (1983) *A Study of the Role and Responsibilities of the Midwife*. Nursing Education Research Unit Report No. 1, Chelsea College, University of London.

Silverman, D. (1972) *The Theory of Organisations*. London: Heinemann.

Stacey, M. (1969) *Methods of Social Research*. Oxford: Pergammon.

7

CARE IN THE COMMUNITY

Jean Davies and Frances Evans

This chapter considers the changing role of the community midwife at a time when nearly all deliveries take place in hospital. During the last two decades midwifery has changed dramatically because of the strength of the ideology that maternity services should be hospital based. The number of community midwives has been reduced and the midwifery profession has become increasingly subsumed in the hospital obstetric team. This change has been poorly documented. In this chapter attention is focused on the role of the community midwife in providing effective antenatal care for women in the community. There are three sections. The first describes the Newcastle Community Midwifery Care Project (the CMC project), the second presents data from the evaluation study of the project and the third discusses the implications of this project and evaluation study for community midwifery as a whole.

THE NEWCASTLE COMMUNITY MIDWIFERY CARE (CMC) PROJECT

Background to the CMC

The CMC project was funded by the Newcastle and Gateshead Inner-City Partnership. It has two aims:

1. To provide enhanced support by midwives to women in their own homes in an area of the city defined as having a concentration of high risk factors.
2. To measure the effects of this intervention on maternal, foetal and infant well-being, consumer satisfaction and the relationships between hospital and community services.

It is hoped that the results of the evaluation study will be taken into account in the future planning of community midwifery across the city.

The CMC project was developed against a background of response to the Second Report from the Social Services Committee on Perinatal and Neonatal Mortality (The Short Report, House of Commons, 1980). This report highlighted the fact that the incidence of low birth weight and perinatal and neonatal deaths is highest among women in the lowest socioeconomic groups. Support for the initiative for the CMC came from the Director of Midwifery and funding for it came from Department of the Environment sources.

It was decided that the project should be located in areas with a high concentration of socioeconomic need and that all women living in these areas should be given enhanced midwifery care by the project midwives. Two areas were selected by reference to data from the 1981 census; these were Cowgate and Newbiggin Hall Estates.

Cowgate and Newbiggin Hall Estates

Cowgate and Newbiggin Hall are both council estates on the edge of the city of Newcastle. Cowgate was built in the 1920s and 1930s and has the potential of being a pleasant estate, having substantial houses, each with its own garden. However, vandalism is rife, there is an air of dereliction, the gardens are untended and many houses are boarded up. There are dogs and dirt everywhere. It has, reputedly, the highest crime rate in the city. There has been a commitment on the part of the local authority to try to upgrade Cowgate, with an intensive local housing management scheme that has prevented the area from becoming completely derelict. Yet the problems have been neither erased nor fully understood. Newbiggin Hall was built later, with blocks of flats as well as houses. It is architecturally poor but the community is recognised as being more stable than that of Cowgate.

The women receiving project care have ranged from a 13-year-old schoolgirl to a 42-year-old woman in her twentieth pregnancy. Single parenting is common, unemployment rates are high and supplementary benefit is the main source of income. Although there are extended family networks on the estates and most residents were born locally, the tenuous quality of community stability became evident when a new family moved into Cowgate from Durham. There was an explosion of violence and residents and local workers came under a state of siege as the family sought to become territorially established. The neighbourhood centre was the focus of attack, with vandalism and theft culminating in an act of arson that closed it for two weeks. Under such conditions of individual and community poverty there are many health hazards for pregnant women. The most obvious are poor nutrition and heavy smoking. More generally, there is a very low level of self-esteem and expectation. The lack of confidence often prevents the pursuit of those activities that could benefit health and well-being and which might alleviate the almost tangible boredom. Despite high male unemployment, women appear to carry the main responsibility for childcare and they often seem to be oppressed within the relationship with their partners. Often, partners are simply not there. At one stage, 22% of the 50 project mothers with partners had their partners either in gaol or awaiting trial.

The CMC project employs four midwives and they work in teams, one to each estate. They cover each other's off-duty and holiday and take turn with the on-call cover for the whole city. In Newbiggin Hall the midwives are based at a health centre, which also houses the child health clinic. In Cowgate, midwives work from the Cowgate neighbourhood centre. This is a converted council house, funded by both the health authority and social services, which aims to provide local, preventive, health and social services. There is a management team of midwives, social workers, local residents and two coordinators who are responsible for the day-to-day running of the centre. The centre is a resource that is welcomed by the many local residents who make use of it, not least because it provides a working telephone on an estate where vandalism is rife! Groups meet there each afternoon and many of these focus on the needs of parents and children. The community midwives hold parentcraft sessions in the centre one afternoon a week and can easily be contacted there at any time. While there are fewer child deliveries in Cowgate than there are in Newbiggin Hall, the midwives in Cowgate have spent much of their time working on the establishment, maintenance and management of the Cowgate neighbour-hood centre, working together with staff from the social services department.

The main emphasis of the project work has been on providing additional ante-natal care. However, continuity of care is given through to the puerperium, and postnatal visits are extended to at least 28 days. Antenatal preparation builds up trust between the woman and her midwife. Every mother is given an in-depth preparation for childbirth and childcare. While this is best achieved in the one-to-one situation at home, mothers can also attend the classes that are held at both of the midwifery bases. Much of the benefit from these lies in the group support that they provide for the women. The classes cover a range of topics, from labour preparation and smoking to nutrition. In Cowgate there are also cooking demon-strations and exercise and swimming sessions.

The midwives have maintained a distinctive record-keeping system, using a 'pa-tient profile'. This records each visit to the woman and notes discussions and observations. It builds up to a full account of a woman's social and medical history, together with a detailed picture of the midwifery management of her pregnancy. At least four antenatal home visits are made, and often more are needed. Antenatal education given on a one-to-one basis in the home is noted on the profile so that a record is kept of the developing curriculum of preparation.

A Midwife's View of the Project

Working on the CMC project is very different from working as a community mid-wife elsewhere in the city. There have been certain difficulties, for example the considerable stresses involved in working in an area of great social and economic deprivation. There has been extensive damage to midwives' cars, although this has become less as time has gone on. There is an acceptance of vandalism and petty theft on the estates, which can be very demoralising to work with. (On one occasion this local criminal 'skill' was welcomed: a project midwife locked her car keys into a car that was 'guaranteed' to be burglar-proof – it took a resident only seconds to effect entry!)

There were also some difficulties involved in working in partnership with social workers. The two professions often have different aims and strategies but, as time has gone on, midwives and social workers have achieved a new co-operation that has enhanced their understanding of one another's different approaches and responsibilities.

A further tension in the work of the project midwives came from the fact of working in an innovative way, different from the rest of the city midwives. Longer established midwives can view change with suspicion and it has taken some time for barriers to be broken down. Overall, one of the most difficult aspects of the project work from the point of view of the midwife has been a less than enthusiastic welcome from the hospital obstetricians.

Despite these difficulties, working on the project has improved job satisfaction for the midwives, who are pleased to have the resources to provide individualised patient care and intensive antenatal education. The style of work is more efficient too, since working in a defined geographical area greatly improves communication. If a woman is out, neighbours and children in the street volunteer information on her whereabouts. News about pregnancies and labours is passed on with amazing speed and midwives are often hailed as they drive around the estates. Increasingly, general health issues are raised and any sight of blood now seems to be thought of as a midwife's province. Midwifery care can be more relevant given in the context of a greater awareness of neighbourhood networks and a well-known local midwife is seen as a person to trust. Several woman are now having their second child in the project and midwives have noticed a marked change in their expectations of care. They are coming to the midwives with early news of pregnancy, often before a visit to the GP. Threatened miscarriages are reported immediately and this is a sign of the trust in which community midwives are now held. In all, the project has had the effect of re-establishing the community midwife as a key local figure and there is no doubt that this has served to improve both job satisfaction and the effectiveness of midwifery care.

The effectiveness of community midwifery care was specifically measured as part of this project by an independent evaluation study. This was carried out by a social scientist on a 3-year appointment, who came into post 8 months after the project work began. In the next section of this chapter the evaluation study is described and certain of its findings relating to antenatal care are presented.

THE EVALUATION STUDY

Several of the characteristics of the CMC project work, as outlined above, make for serious methodological difficulties in the project's evaluation. Such difficulty is a recurrent theme in the literature dealing with community health programmes (Fenton-Lewis and Modle, 1982; Beattie, 1984). In this project the emphases on quality of care and education for prevention are difficult to quantify, and clinical outcomes such as perinatal mortality cannot be tested for statistical significance because the numbers involved are too small. This evaluation overcame such difficulties by using both qualitative and quantitative techniques. Four methods were used, which are described below.

Case Note Survey

The case note survey is a strictly quantitative measurement of health outcome based on data extracted from hospital notes. Data recorded include: maternal weight; maternal height; social and medical history at booking; clinic attendance; child birth weight; and gestational age.

The first study population for the case note survey consisted of all women resident in the project area who booked in for antenatal care between October 1984 and October 1985. In all there were 263 bookings. A second study population consisted of controls for this group. These women lived in parts of the city with broadly similar socioeconomic characteristics to the project areas and were matched to the project mothers in terms of age, parity, social class, marital status, hospital booking and type of antenatal care. Two further, retrospective, study populations were constructed. One consisted of women who were resident in the project areas and had given birth during the year preceding the onset of intervention. The second was made up of women in the control areas who gave birth in that year, and these were matched to the retrospective case group. In total, over 800 notes were reviewed in this case note survey.

Survey of Client Opinion

This was the most time-consuming aspect of the evaluation. All women living in the project area who booked for antenatal care between October 1984 and October 1985 were interviewed twice, once antenatally and once postnatally. A total of 222 project mothers were interviewed antenatally and 198 were seen postnatally. Questionnaires focused on women's behaviour (for example in terms of clinic attendance and eating, drinking and smoking patterns), their opinions about the maternity services and their socioeconomic environment. Throughout the questionnaires there was an emphasis on qualitative perspectives and, in particular, women were repeatedly asked to explain their behaviour and speak freely about their ratings of the maternity services. A control group of mothers was also interviewed. This was the group described as the second study population in the case note survey above, i.e. women living in the parts of the city with no midwifery intervention who were matched to the project mothers in terms of age, parity, social class, marital status, hospital booking and type of antenatal care. All interviews took place in the women's own homes.

Time Budget Study

This study quantified midwives' time so as to be able accurately to describe how project midwives' time was spent and to demonstrate how this is different from the work of other community midwives. The four project midwives and nine midwives working in the control area were asked to keep a detailed diary of time use for a week. Research observation before the study week had enabled a coded list of activities to be compiled and these were used by the midwives in recording their work.

Staff Survey

Qualitative data were collected from hospital and community staff by diverse means. Individual, tape-recorded interviews were held with all project midwives and with all hospital consultants in the division of obstetrics and gynaecology. A postal questionnaire was administered to all other community midwives and to GPs who

Table 7.1 Frequency of antenatal home visits by community midwives

Number of visits	Percentage of all project cases (n = 198)	Percentage of all controls (n = 184)
0	1.0	5.4
1	2.5	62.0
2,3	18.7	26.1
4,5	26.3	4.9
6–10	28.8	1.1
11–20	14.1	0.0
21+	8.1	0.5
	$p < 0.001$	

had project mothers in their practice. Interviews were held at the four GP surgeries based on the estates. One-off written queries were made to other professionals who had contact with the project.

Findings

The data set collected by the methods above was vast, but discussion will be limited to those parts of it that relate to the role of the community midwife in the antenatal period. Three main outcome measures are presented: antenatal education; client opinion; and diet and smoking behaviour.

Antenatal Education

The data demonstrated the extent of antenatal education, both inside and outside the home. Having fewer clients enabled project midwives to have the time to make far more antenatal home visits than did midwives in the control area (Table 7.1). These extra visits enabled project midwives to carry out effective home-based education, which could be given in the context of a growing relationship between themselves and their clients. Because of the additional resources project midwives were able to cover a far wider range of topics than was possible in the control area (Table 7.2).

Because midwives were familiar with the home circumstances of women, they were able to give individualised education that was targetted at the special needs of

Table 7.2 Content and extent of antenatal home education

Content of education	Percentage of all project cases (n = 198)	Percentage of all controls (n = 184)
Infant feeding	60.1	15.2
Contraception	36.8	2.1
Eating	43.9	2.7
Drinking	20.2	2.7
Smoking	40.9	9.8
Baby care	23.2	2.2

Table 7.3 Rating of antenatal community midwifery care

Rating	Percentage of all cases (n = 198)	Percentage of all controls (n = 184)
1 Very satisfied	72.2	35.3
2 Satisfied	19.2	41.3
3 Indifferent	3.5	12.0
4 Dissatisfied	3.5	6.5
5 Very dissatisfied	0.5	1.1
Don't know, etc.	1.0	3.8

each woman. In particular, it was possible to give advice that was pertinent for women with considerable socioeconomic disadvantage.

Outside the home antenatal parentcraft classes were held by project midwives and they had more time than would be usual to recruit women to such classes and to follow up defaulters. Attendance at classes was dramatically increased by the midwifery intervention. Thirty-one per cent of project cases, compared with only 6% of controls, went to some classes and this shows a sharp increase from the most recent previous pregnancy, when only 4% of cases and 3% of controls attended.

Client Opinion

The survey of mothers showed clearly that women preferred this style of midwifery care to that available elsewhere in the city. They were asked to rate their satisfaction with community midwifery care in the antenatal period on a scale from 1 (very satisfied) to 5 (very dissatisfied), and Table 7.3 shows that satisfaction levels were extremely high.

Data collected from women who had had a previous pregnancy showed that project mothers were far more likely than were control mothers to feel that their antenatal community midwifery care had improved since their most recent previous pregnancy (Table 7.4).

Qualitative data collected during the interviews gave a vivid account of how much the project mothers enjoyed their care. Much of what they said highlighted their need for support and emphasised their appreciation of the one-to-one relationship:

'It's marvellous, it's someone to talk to, to keep an interest in you. Even if no-one else is.'

'At the time my mam was away, and I was glad of the company I had off the midwife.'

'I was very satisfied, she was marvellous; it's like talking to your mother, talking to her. She was dead canny, really smashing.'

Table 7.4 Retrospective comparison of antenatal community midwifery care

Rating	Percentage of cases with previous pregnancy (n = 107)	Percentage of controls with previous pregnancy (n = 105)
Better	89.7	27.6
The same	9.3	68.6
Worse	0.9	2.8

Table 7.5   Changes in diet in the study and previous pregnancies

	Cases (%)	Controls (%)
Study pregnancy	n = 198	n = 184
Changes made	63.6	66.8
No changes made	36.3	33.1
Previous pregnancy	n = 127	n = 118
Changes made	48.1	65.2
No changes made	51.9	34.7

Diet and Smoking Behaviour

The project intervention had an effect on diet during pregnancy in several ways. First, a far higher proportion of project mothers changed their diet during the study pregnancy than they had in their previous pregnancy, whereas in the control group, the proportion making dietary changes remained the same (Table 7.5).

Second, case mothers were more likely than control mothers to modify their diet in order to improve their health.

Third, 11% of case mothers, compared with 1% of control group mothers, were still eating fewer sweet foods at the time of the postnatal interviews than they were before intervention.

The study demonstrates that many mothers in the project group had an inadequate diet and it highlighted the need to focus antenatal education on this area. For example, 40% of project mothers ate no green vegetables or fruit during the day preceding the antenatal interview and a further 36% ate only one or two portions. Eighty-one per cent ate no wholegrain foods during that day, and 67% ate three or more portions of chips, white bread, shop bought pie or pasty or frosted breakfast cereal.

The intervention affected smoking behaviour in two ways. First, more cases than controls cut down or gave up smoking. Analysis of the smoking data by social class showed that the effect of the midwifery intervention was particulary marked among women whose head of household was unemployed. In the case group 47% of such women stopped or cut down smoking during pregnancy, compared with 25% in the control group. It should be remembered that women in households relying on supplementary benefit are under extreme stress during pregnancy and would be expected to increase smoking as a response to stress. The fact that the reverse was true is evidence that antenatal education was successfully targetted at those women who were particularly socioeconomically disadvantaged.

DISCUSSION AND CONCLUSION

The evaluation of the CMC project demonstrates that this style of community midwifery is effective in that it focuses antenatal care where it is needed and greatly enhances client satisfaction. The project as a whole has re-established the importance of the midwife in the community and has emphasised her role in the antenatal period.

It is clear that much of this antenatal work is of a preventive nature, and its long-term benefits may prove to be as significant as are the short-term outcome measures such as parentcraft attendance, client satisfaction and diet and smoking patterns. The experience of project midwives has suggested that their antenatal work has only been so successful because it is done in the woman's own environment in the local community on a one-to-one basis. Contact with midwives is easy and acceptable when they have a high local profile. In the home it is possible for the midwife to concentrate on aspects of the woman's individual needs that cannot be dealt with either in a group situation where shyness may inhibit or in clinics where there is simply not enough time or space.

Intensive antenatal care also has benefits for the postnatal period. Visiting is qualitatively different and problems such as postnatal depression can be more easily identified in a patient who is already well known to the midwife. Working with restricted resources elsewhere in the city, community midwives are aware of the routinisation of postnatal visits and their forced superficiality. Project resources have enabled more meaningful postnatal care, which has grown from the antenatal input, during which mother and midwife were able to build up a trusting relationship.

The evaluation study demonstrates that working class Newcastle-upon-Tyne mothers were extremely satisfied with this style of midwifery care. In particular, they valued the quality of the one-to-one relationship with the midwife. The midwives themselves felt that the success of this relationship lay in the opportunity to spend time with women in their own homes. This exposed a more complex and multi-dimensional picture of a woman than is possible in a clinic, and a clear picture of her and her pregnancy was built up. Women felt more comfortable with care given in the context of their lives as a whole and this in turn enhanced their confidence in motherhood.

Thus the CMC project has demonstrated the effectiveness of enhanced community midwifery and highlighted the need for intensive antenatal input. This is an important finding at a time when the role of the community midwife has changed as a result of the move to hospital confinements. There has been a radical alteration in childbirth in this country as it has become increasingly institutionalised, moving away from the communities in which the babies will be raised. The emphasis on the physical and medical aspects of pregnancy has become stronger, whereas that on its social and psychological aspects has weakened (Oakley, 1979, 1980). Measurements of indices such as weight gain and urine content have become standardised but a holistic approach to pregnancy has become impossible as care has been fragmented. Increasingly, the midwife has been seen as an assistant to the doctor, carrying out certain clinical measurements but leaving the consultation to the GP or obstetrician. There has been a consistent undermining of the midwife's former responsibility for the care of normal pregnancy and maternity care has become more and more based on the expectation of pathology than of normality.

The project has demonstrated that these fundamental changes in the midwife's role are not irreversible. Working in the community with adequate resources to provide intensive antenatal care enables the development of a midwifery style that was perhaps more common a generation ago. Older midwives have commented that the project work echoes their own training, when the community midwife was a trusted figure in the local community. Such midwives have seen their professional status diminished during their working lives, but the project has enabled a new enhancement of the midwifery role at a time when many see it to be under a serious threat.

Research can be an instrument of change and it is hoped that the CMC project will show the way for change both in Newcastle-upon-Tyne and elsewhere in the country. This style of working has met the needs of an extremely disadvantaged urban population as well as those of the community midwife. Such work should be seen primarily as an investment and one that may yield substantial rewards in both the short and the long term. The investment is three fold: in the personal and social development of working class, inner-city women; in the health of the next generation on the city estates; and in the future of the midwifery profession. All three are areas in which investment is urgently needed and it is hoped that the material presented in this chapter will encourage debate about the establishment of more community midwifery initiatives such as this around the country.

REFERENCES

Beattie, A. (1984) *Evaluating Community Health Initiatives*. Paper for NCVO/LUSC Conference. London: Kings Fund Centre.

Fenton-Lewis, A. and Modle, W.J. (1982) Health indicators: what are they? *Health Trends*, **145**: 3–8.

House of Commons (1980) *Second Report from the Social Services Committee on Perinatal and Neonatal Mortality* (Chairman: Short). London: HMSO.

Oakley, A. (1979) *Becoming a Mother*. Oxford: Martin Robertson.

Oakley, A. (1980) *Women Confined*. Oxford: Martin Robertson.

8

ANTENATAL EDUCATION

Tricia Murphy-Black and Ann Faulkner

Antenatal education within the National Health Service (NHS) developed from two separate traditions: the preparation for childbirth and the hygiene traditions. It has been demonstrated in both that: attendance at classes remains poor (Boyd and Sellars, 1982; Royal College of Midwives, 1966); the physical benefits are variable and depend on the training (Burnett, 1956; Roberts et al, 1953); the involvement of fathers is limited (McCabe et al, 1984); the classes do not meet the information needs of individuals (Chamberlain, 1975); and the teaching is poor (Taylor, 1985). It can be asked whether or not the aims of either tradition are met and whether or not the classes serve any useful purpose.

Two major papers from the government, the Court (Department of Health and Social Security, 1976) and the Short Reports (House of Commons, 1980), expressed the view that antenatal education was generally seen as being beneficial for parents but that there was little evidence to support this opinion. The Maternity Services Advisory Committee (1982), set up in response to the Short Report, produced guidelines for health authorities. Concerning the educational preparation of women it stated:

> 'Classes should be arranged at times and in places which are convenient for as many as possible, but for groups of a size which permit discussion and participation by all present. The content and method of presentation should be reviewed regularly by midwives and health visitors together, taking into account the contribution that other professionals might make, so that the maximum benefit is obtained for local needs.'

Although some of the problems identified in antenatal education may stem from the organisation of the classes, much rests with the teacher. Teachers should be able to meet the needs of the mothers attending classes, and this may indicate that there is a need for them to shift to learner-centered teaching rather than having a set 8-week course with specific information to impart, irrespective of how much the mothers may know already.

Midwives and health visitors have long accepted their health education role. Health visitors, especially, are providers of advice and education (Royal College of Nursing, 1983). There is some specific, if limited, training for both groups for this role (Jones and Barnes, 1985a,b; Royal College of Midwives Scottish Board, 1986). Training for the teaching role is needed, especially for midwives, despite general agreement that midwives should teach (Sweet, 1984). Those who do not have formal training learn by 'sitting next to Nelly' or by basing it on their own experience. Until recently, training at both basic and post-basic levels was towards lecture-based teaching, with the teacher making the decisions. This is the only role model the antenatal teachers have had. Yet this style of teaching could be intimidating when dealing with emotional topics and could prevent discussion that allows mothers to air their fears and learn from each other. Health visitors are in a slightly better position than are midwives as their training includes health education but they still need training in groupwork skills (Perkins and Morris, 1979).

Despite the doubt expressed about the value of antenatal education and the reasons for its support by the government, there are compelling reasons for not only continuing with antenatal education but also making it as effective as possible. Problems with the communication skills of nurses and the maternity services have been identified. A possible means of improving antenatal education to make it effective is by improving the teaching, groupwork and communication skills of the midwives and health visitors who are involved in providing this service. Although there are other courses for prospective parents, such as those provided by the National Childbirth Trust and the active birth movement, these are private and a fee is charged. It is only within the NHS that there is no direct charge, which is important considering that the group in greatest need of discussing the skills and life-style options are the socially disadvantaged. Antenatal education should appeal to these parents and it might do so if classes are presented as attractive and inviting and if the teaching is stimulating and satisfying.

There is a need to help those who are worried by pregnancy, unsure of what childbirth entails and unaware of the demands of parenthood (Perkins, 1979). The benefits of antenatal education, Perkins (1979) argues, are the help in adjustment to pregnancy and parenthood, in how to use the services of professional staff and in how to cope with labour and learn the practical skills of baby care. Antenatal education could be seen as the 'shop window' not only of maternity services but also of other services. For the young girl whose first independent contact with health-care officialdom may be during her first pregnancy, this is a vital contact. If this contact is a good one, and if subsequent contacts reinforce that the welfare services do, in fact, have her welfare at heart, she may be in a position to seek help before reaching breaking point – the breaking point that may end in the non-accidental injury or death of her child.

On this basis it is worth the effort to produce effective changes in antenatal education. These changes will have to concentrate on making existing provision better known in order to improve attendance. As the audience needs to be attract-ed the 'school' image should be replaced by a more informal one; the needs of parents have to be met. This may involve many variations within one geographical area. The changes in society will have to be reflected to allow for the many life-styles imposed by our multicultural population, and a more individual and flexible approach is required. The teaching needs to be pitched at a level that will not discourage those who attend but will encourage them to discuss aspects of parent-hood that are uppermost in their minds. To achieve this the teachers need to be confident in their teaching skills and abilities to establish and keep a group together.

STUDY METHODS

Following research of the local antenatal education service in Nottinghamshire, a training course was devised by Perkins and Craig (1981) and used with midwives and health visitors. This course was run in two other parts of the country. An evaluation of the course was funded by the Health Education Council and was undertaken in these two centres.

The teaching and group skills training course, originally consisting of 5 half days, was expanded to a full week. Details of the course and its development are published in Murphy-Black and Faulkner (1988). The material common to both centres comprised sessions on teaching and groupwork skills. The material added to the Perkins and Craig course consisted of further aspects of teaching theory, communications and reports of local research in the centres. Centre A had sessions on how to teach relaxation and exercises and centre B had 'update on midwifery' sessions.

The groupwork skills material emphasised making antenatal classes informal and welcoming so that the women attending would feel that they could participate and would be encouraged to talk about their concerns. Much of the training course was experimental. The midwives and health visitors learnt how it felt to join a group and practical ways of making a group 'gel'. These antenatal teachers spent time in small groups where they discussed issues, tried out techniques that they had just learnt and contributed to the course from their own experience. Details such as using first names, seating arrangements, provision of a cup of tea and wearing uniform were discussed and, where appropriate, tried out. Both centres had a session near the end of the course with mothers attending, so that the midwives and health visitors could use techniques of teaching and questioning that they had learnt during the course.

The evaluation of the course consisted of two studies: a questionnaire study and an observation study. There were seven questionnaires – one pre-course, five during the course and one post-course – administered to the 65 midwives and health visitors attending the courses in the two centres. The results of the questionnaire study are reported in Black (1985).

The observation study involved 23 midwives and health visitors teaching in 76 antenatal classes. Twenty-three sessions were observed before and 53 after the teachers attended the training course. The methods used were:

1. *Interaction analysis*: the live recording of the verbal aspects of teaching behaviour, using an adaptation of Flanders' (1970) categories for interaction analysis.
2. *Checklist*: the recording of environmental and physical aspects of the class, including those that could and could not be altered by the teacher.
3. *Description*: a subjective description of the class, which noted the behaviour of all those present in the class and any features that could have an influence on the class.

Interaction Analysis

Diers and Leonard (1966) define interaction analysis as:

'the description of the content and structure of communication between people, [which] provides the means of specifying, quantifying and hence communicating to others the components of different kinds of nursing process.'

Interaction analysis has been used for observation in social situations, such as in groups, in schools and by nurses. Nurse–patient interaction has been observed; for instance, the home visits of public health nurses to their patients were analysed by Conant (1965). Johnson (1964) and Kerrigan (1957) analysed conversations between student nurses and patients. Reynolds and Cormack (1985) described the frequency and content of individual contributions in group dynamics. Kishi (1983) studied the communication patterns between health-care providers and clients at a well-baby clinic, and Vehvilainen (1984) observed the interaction between midwives and mothers in labour, both researchers using Flanders' (1970) categories.

Flanders Interaction Analysis Categories (FIAC)

FIAC was devised:

'to develop more objective techniques for analyzing interaction, techniques which not only provide evidence of change, but also become a stepping stone to a systematic inquiry into . . . teaching behavior.'

It is not always possible to measure teacher behaviour by pupil achievement (McNeil and Popham, 1973) as there may be a wide range of pupil attitudes. FIAC, however, is a means of describing the interaction between the teacher and the class.

The 10 categories described by Flanders (1970) consist of seven to measure teacher initiation and response, two for pupil initiation and response and one for silence and confusion. FIAC measures a specific chain of events, which can be analysed to demonstrate which patterns are associated with effective teaching. Flanders (1970) affirmed that:

'Teaching behavior, by its very nature, exists in a context of social interaction. The acts of teaching lead to reciprocal contacts between the teacher and the pupils, and the interchange itself is called teaching.'

Flanders gave two reasons for examining classroom interaction:

1. To identify patterns of teaching.
2. To gain knowledge of the differences in educational outcomes associated with teaching.

The focus is on teaching behaviour and its relationship to classroom interaction.

The concepts used by Flanders, which underpin the development of his interaction analysis categories are:

'1. classroom interaction refers to a chain of events which occur one after the other, each occupying only a segment of time;
2. teaching behaviour has been defined as acts by the teacher which occur in the context of classroom interaction;
3. an event is the shortest possible act that a trained observer can identify and record;
4. a pattern is a short chain of events that can be identified, occurs frequently enough to be of interest, and can be given a label.'

FIAC was originally designed as a research tool but Flanders later used it as a means of training student teachers.

The major feature of this category system is in the analysis of initiative and response. This was one of the reasons for choosing the system for this study, as the aim of the training course was to encourage the antenatal teachers to use the ideas and feelings that come from mothers in the class. The FIAC system was adapted for this study; adaptability is one of the advantages that Flanders (1970) claims for his system, and it has been modified by others.

THE SAMPLE

The course in centre B, which was organised jointly by four health authorities, had 37 attenders. As the single health authority centre A had smaller numbers in the courses, two courses were evaluated to increase the numbers (12 people on course A1 and 16 on A2). Initial analysis demonstrated there were no statistical differences between A1 and A2, so they were combined for comparison with centre B.

The sample described here comprises the 62 (94.4%) subjects who returned the pre-course questionnaire, 65 of which had been distributed. Chi square tests demonstrated no statistically significant differences between the centres (A and B) and the occupational groups (midwives and health visitors) for the length of service and teaching experience before the course, as shown in Table 8.1.

The majority of respondents (40.3%) had started antenatal teaching since 1979, although six did not give any information on this. Of the nine who had been teaching since 1973, there were twice as many in centre B as centre A and twice as many health visitors as midwives. Antenatal classes were taught either on a regular or part-time basis or as occasional sessions.

The two factors that showed differences at a level that was possibly significant were:

1. the incidence of previous training in teaching skills;
2. the decision-making process for attending the course.

Table 8.1 Profile of the subjects in centres A and B

Centre	A (n = 26)	B (n = 36)	Total (n = 62)	Percentage
Midwives	11	16	27	43.5
Health visitors	15	20	35	56.5
Length of service				
Not answered	1	4	5	8.1
1–5 years	19	21	40	64.5
6–10 years	3	7	10	16.1
>11 years	3	4	7	11.3
Previous teaching experience				
Yes	20	31	51	82.3
No	6	5	11	17.7

There were 15 subjects (24.2%) who had some training relevant to antenatal education. Only three of the 27 midwives had training for their teaching role, compared with over a third of the health visitors; these differences were possibly significant at $p = 0.06$ level.

Information about the decision to attend the course was sought, with the following options given to the subjects:

1. It was suggested by a senior member of staff.
2. You asked to be sent.
3. You decided yourself.

Those who answered (2) or (3) or a combination of these were included in the category 'self-selected', whereas those who replied (1) were designated 'manager selected'. Centre B had significantly more ($p = 0.004$) respondents who said that this decision was made at the suggestion of a senior member of staff. This difference was not apparent between the occupations (Figure 8.1).

There were 23 subjects observed teaching 76 antenatal classes. There were no statistically significant differences in the characteristics of the teachers from the centres A and B, the occupational groups (midwives and health visitors) or the incidence of pre- and post-course teaching.

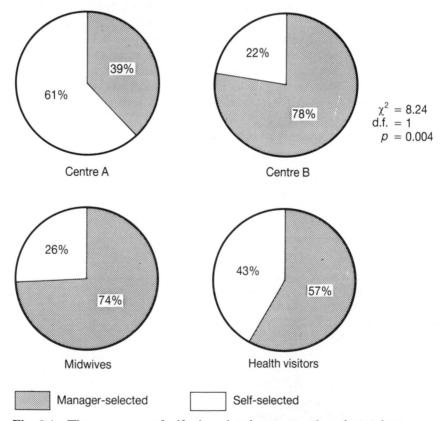

Fig. 8.1 The percentage of self-selected and manager-selected attenders

Table 8.2 The distribution of the 76 sessions between centres, occupations, place of teaching, single or team teaching and pre- and post-course

	Number	Percentage
Centre A	29	38.2
Centre B	47	61.8
Midwives	32	42.1
Health visitors	44	57.9
Health centres/clinics	57	75.0
Hospital	18	23.7
GP unit	1	1.3
Single teacher	42	55.3
Team teaching	34	44.7
Pre-course	23	30.3
Post-course	53	69.7

Table 8.2 shows that there was an imbalance in the amount of observation pre-course (23 sessions) and post-course (56 sessions) owing to factors outside the control of the evaluator. There were no statistical differences in the other factors listed in Table 8.2.

DATA COLLECTION

The observation took place in the health centres or hospitals in which the midwives and health visitors normally held their classes. The observer sat just outside the group and transcribed the speech of teachers and mothers into the Flanders categories, recording them on a data collection sheet held on a clipboard. The categories were recorded at 3-second intervals throughout the class, excluding any films, videos and relaxation and exercise periods.

ANALYSIS AND RESULTS

Flanders (1970) gives detailed instructions for the analysis of the data obtained from observation in the classroom. The procedure involves:

1. calculating the length of observation;
2. calculating the percentage of teacher talk, pupil talk and silence or confusion. Teacher talk in the Flanders categories involves the categories designated 1–7, pupil talk is in categories 8–9, while silence or confusion is in category 10. In this study the adapted categories were collapsed back into the 10 original categories for analysis;
3. calculating the eight ratios proposed by Flanders.

Flanders' eight ratios are:

1. *Teacher Response Ratio (TRR)*: 'an index which corresponds to the teacher's tendency to react to ideas and feeling of the pupils.'
2. *Teacher Question Ratio (TQR)*: 'an index representing the tendency of a teacher to use questions when guiding the more content oriented part of the class discussion . . . it will vary as the teacher solicits pupil reactions to ideas which the teacher considers important or checks on understanding by asking questions.'
3. *Pupil Initiation Ratio (PIR)*: 'to indicate what proportion of pupil talk was judged by the observer to be an act of initiation.'
4. *Instantaneous Teacher Response Ratio (TRR89)*: 'the tendency of the teacher to praise or integrate pupil ideas and feelings into the class discussion, at the moment the pupils stop talking.'
5. *Instantaneous Teacher Question Ratio (TQR89)*: 'the tendency of the teacher to respond to pupil talk with questions based on his own ideas, compared with his tendency to lecture.'
6. *Content Cross Ratio (CCR)*: 'those statements which are least likely to be involved with problems of reward and punishment, reacting to the ideas and feeling of the pupil and giving of assignments and direction, as these are not classified in the categories 4 and 5.'
7. *Steady State Ratio (SSR)*: 'reflects the tendency of teacher and pupil talk to remain in the same category for periods longer than 3 seconds. The higher this ratio, the less rapid is the interchange between the teacher and the pupils.'
8. *Pupil Steady State Ratio (PSSR)*: 'a more sensitive index to the rapidity of teacher–pupil interchange when the amount of pupil talk is average or above average.'

The most appropriate statistical test of significance for the ratios was the non-parametric Mann-Whitney U test, as not all the ratios were normally distributed.

The profile data from the pre-course questionnaire (see Figure 8.1 above) had demonstrated that there were significantly more subjects from centre B who attended the course at the suggestion of their managers than were self-selected. This was supported in the reasons given for attending the course, with 13 subjects from centre B commenting that they were 'sent on the course'.

Of the 76 classes observed there was information about the decision-making process for the teachers of 71 of the classes. This information was not available when the subset was chosen for inclusion in the observation study. There were 16 classes taught by the self-selected teachers and 55 by the manager-selected teachers; these were analysed to determine whether or not there were any differences in the pre- and post-course levels of interaction.

Figure 8.2 shows the percentages of mother and teacher talk and silence in the two groups. There was a significant increase in mother talk and a significant decrease in teacher talk in the self-selected group post-course. The significant decrease in the proportion of silence post-course in the manager-selected group was associated (but not at a significant level) with an increase in teacher talk and a decrease in mother talk.

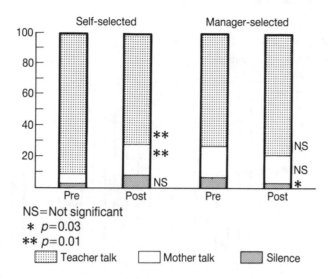

Fig. 8.2 The percentage of mother talk, teacher talk and silence in the classes taught by the self-selected group and the manager-selected group, pre- and post-course

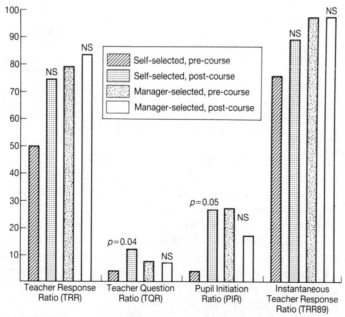

Fig. 8.3 The Teacher Response Ratio, Teacher Question Ratio, Pupil Initiation Ratio and Instantaneous Teacher Response Ratio in the classes taught by the self-selected group and the manager-selected group, pre- and post-course

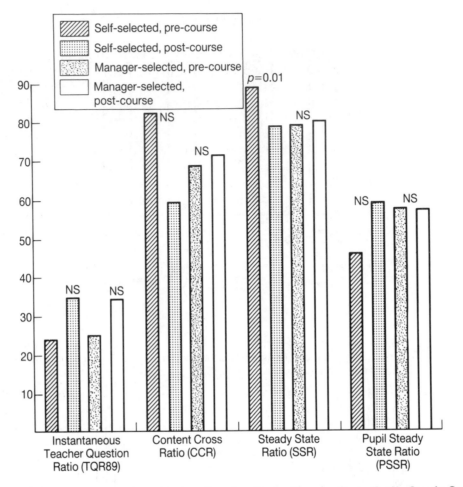

Fig. 8.4 The Instantaneous Teacher Question Ratio, Content Cross Ratio, Steady State Ratio and Pupil Steady State Ratio in the classes taught by the self-selected group and the manager-selected group, pre- and post-course

Neither group demonstrated any difference in the TRR (Figure 8.3), but the self-selected teachers increased their use of questions to guide the content-orientated part of the discussion (TQR). The self-selected group had a significant increase in the initiation by the mothers in their post-course classes, whereas this measure decreased in the classes taught by the manager-selected group. The increase in the instantaneous response to the mothers' ideas was not significant in the self-selected teachers and did not reach the level maintained by the manager-selected group.

Both groups had a post-course increase in the use of questions in response to the mothers' talk (Figure 8.4), but not at a significant level. The self-selected group put less emphasis on content post-course, whereas there was a slight increase in emphasis by the manager-selected group. There was a significant decrease in the SSR post-course, which indicated a more rapid interchange between teacher and mothers in the classes taught by the self-selected group.

DISCUSSION

The antenatal classes observed, when examined as a whole, demonstrated that the teachers talked for about four-fifths of the class, the mothers contributed to less than one-fifth and the remainder of the time was spent in silence or confusion. The teachers responded to the mothers' ideas and feelings but did not use questions to guide the content. The amount of discussion that the mothers initiated was low, but when the mothers did introduce their ideas they were praised or their ideas were integrated into the discussion. About one third of the teachers' responses to mothers' talk were questions based on the teachers' ideas. There was a high level of emphasis on the class content. The interchange between mother and teacher was quite high, although the low level of mother talk may have given a spuriously high result.

Differences in the levels of interaction between teachers and mothers were mainly in the classes taught by the small group of self-selected teachers. This group had lower levels of interaction pre-course and the post-course observation demonstrated that they had achieved higher levels than had the manager-selected group (Table 8.3).

For both measures (mother talk and PIR), the manager-selected group had higher levels pre-course than had the self-selected group. The pre-course levels of the self-selected group were lower than the means for all the pre-course classes. Despite this small amount of interaction initially, the group improved significantly and in the post-course results had higher levels than the manager-selected group. Although not at a statistically significant level, there was a reduction in the mothers' involvement in the post-course classes taught by the manager-selected group.

When the 10 measures of interaction (see pp. 82) were examined, the self-selected group had a significant difference in five measures post-course. Their teaching produced classes where the mothers talked more and the teachers less. They used more questions to guide the content or solicit the mothers' reactions to the teachers' ideas. There was an increase in the proportion of the class in which the mothers initiated the content or matter for discussion. A reduction in the SSR indicated that there was an increased interchange between teachers and mothers, implying that these teachers did not dominate the classes.

The other six measures also indicate an increased interaction, although not reaching levels of statistical significance. The self-selected group responded more to mothers' ideas or feelings, which they were more likely to praise or integrate into the

Table 8.3 The mean percentage of mother talk and the pupil (mother) initiation ratio (PIR) in the pre- and post-course classes taught by the self-selected group and the manager-selected group

Selection	Percentage of mother talk		PIR	
	Pre	Post	Pre	Post
Self	5.2	20.6	3.8	26.6
Manager	19.7	17.9	27.2	16.9
All classes	16.6	17.5	22.2	17.9

discussion. There was an increased use of questions rather than lecture when responding to mother talk and a decrease in emphasis on the content. As the amount of mother talk was above average, the increased PSSR indicated a rapid interchange between mothers and teachers.

In contrast, the post-course classes of the manager-selected group demonstrated less interaction than did the pre-course classes, although for most measures this did not reach statistically significant levels. The mothers talked less and the teachers more; there was significantly less time spent in silence. There was a slight increase in the response to mothers' ideas and feelings but no change in the pattern of questioning or use of mothers' ideas. Mothers initiated fewer discussions in the post-course classes, and there was an increase in the use of lecturing and reduced interchange between mother and teacher.

Possible explanations for these differences have been sought by examining characteristics of the self-selected group. Three of the five pre-course classes were on teaching baby bathing (the overall percentage of talk of the 13 mothers for these classes was the lowest in the topic grouping, at 10.4%), which may have contributed to the low mother talk percentage in the self-selected group pre-course. The PIR, however, in baby bathing was higher than in antenatal and labour topics and the fathers' classes, so the relevance of the baby bathing topics to the low interaction level in the self-selected group is not clear. There was an equal distribution of all topics among the post-course classes taught by the self-selected group.

The time of post-course observation was similar for the whole group (ranging from 5 to 9 months for the self-selected group and 4 to 10 months for all post-course observations). Four of the pre-course and 7 of the post-course classes were taught in teams.

The 16 classes taught by the self-selected group consisted of 11 teachers, of whom 9 were from centre A and 2 from centre B. The proportion of self-selected subjects in the whole sample was 61.5% in centre A and 22.2% in centre B. The division of occupation of the self-selected group in the observation study was two midwives and nine health visitors. Eight subjects, including both the midwives, had previous experience of teaching and three, all health visitors, had previous training in teaching. This would appear to indicate that self-selection to the course was dependent on the group's own perceptions of their teaching ability rather than on experience, training or occupation. These pre-course results seem to demonstrate that this group were accurate in their assessment of their own teaching skills, as their pre-course teaching was associated with low levels of interaction.

The interaction results may indicate that the manager-selected group did not feel a need for further training for their teaching role. As their pre-course levels of interaction were higher than those of the self-selected group, there may be some justification for this judgment. The post-course results demonstrate, however, that their interaction improved only very slightly and did not reach the levels achieved by the self-selected group post-course. As the self-selected group, even post-course, did not have classes with as much mother talk as pupil talk as in other studies – for example 40% and 52% in Amidon and Giammatteo's (1967) study and 51.8% reported by Wagner (1973) – this improvement is still only a small one.

The other comparisons of the pre- and post-course differences in interaction revealed little change. Comparison between centres and the classes led by midwives and health visitors showed either no or only a small amount of increase in inter-action. In the nine classes that were matched pre- and post-course for teacher, topics and place of teaching, there were no differences. There was an increased percentage of mother talk, a high ratio of initiation of the mothers' ideas and a rapid interchange with the teachers in the breast feeding classes. The baby bathing classes were associated with reduced interaction between mother and teacher as there was an increase in the percentage of teacher talk, reduced response from the teacher to the mothers' ideas and less integration into the discussion. When babies were included in the class, the percentage of teacher talk was reduced as was the teachers' response to the mothers' ideas; there was an increase in the mothers' initiation of ideas but a reduction of praise or integration of ideas into the discussion and reaction to ideas and feeling of the mothers.

CONCLUSION

Although the overall levels of interaction between teachers and mothers in antenatal classes were low in the classes observed, the teachers who wanted to attend the teaching and groupwork skills training course were those whose post-course teach-ing demonstrated increased interaction between mother and teacher. Where poss-ible, the staff chosen to attend such a course should be those who themselves perceive a need for further training. If there are staff who are unwilling to attend such a training course, consideration should be given to helping them to become aware of their own needs for development. Evaluation of their own classes may be one such means.

One method of increasing interaction between mothers and teachers, which could easily be used, is the inclusion of a mother with her baby in all antenatal classes. This may cause disruption to the class if the baby is fretful. However, the advantages gained from such a topic of conversation will overcome the possible disadvantages. Babies are frequently a stimulus to conversation.

REFERENCES

Amidon, E. and Giammatteo, M. (1967) The verbal behaviour of superior elementary teach-ers. In: *Interaction Analysis: Theory, Research and Application*, Amidon, E. and Hough, J.B. (eds.). London: Addison-Wesley.

Boyd, C. and Sellars, L. (1982) *The British Way of Birth*. London: Pan.

Burnett, C.W.F. (1956) The value of antenatal exercises. *Journal of Obstetrics and Gynaecol-ogy*, **63**: 40–57.

Chamberlain, G. (1975) Antenatal education: the consumer's view. *Midwife, Health Visitor and Community Nurse*, **11**: 289–922.

Conant, L.H. (1965) Use of Bales' interaction process anlaysis to study nurse–patient inter-action. *Nursing Research*, **14**: 304–309.

Department of Health and Social Security, Committee for Child Health Services (1976) *Fit for the Future* (Chairman: Court). London: HMSO.

Diers, D. and Leonard, R.C. (1966) Interaction analysis in nursing research. *Nursing Research*, **15**: 225–228.

Flanders, N.A. (1970) *Analyzing Teaching Behaviour*. Reading, Massachusetts: Addison-Wesley.

House of Commons (1980) *Second Report of the Social Services Committee on Perinatal and Neonatal Mortality* (Chairman: Short). London: HMSO.

Johnson, B.S. (1964) Relationships between verbal patterns of nursing students and therapeutic effectiveness. *Nursing Research*, **13**: 339–342.

Jones, P. and Barnes, D. (1985a) Health visitors as group leaders. *Midwife, Health Visitor and Community Nurse*, **21**: 396–404.

Jones, P. and Barnes, D. (1985b) Listening to mother. *Nursing Times*, **81**(13): 46.

Kerrigan, M.R. (1957) Analysis of conversations between selected students and their assigned patients. *Nursing Research*, **6**: 43–45.

Kishi, K.I. (1983) Communication patterns of health teaching and information recall. *Nursing Research*, **32**: 230–235.

McCabe, F., Rocheron, Y., Dickson, R. and McCron, R. (1984) Antenatal education in primary care: a survey of general practitioners, midwives and health visitors. Leicester: Centre for Mass Communication Research, University of Leicester.

Maternity Services Advisory Committee (1982) *Maternity Care in Action, Part 1: Antenatal Care* (Chairman: Munro). London: HMSO.

Murphy-Black, T. and Faulkner, A. (1988) *Antenatal Group Skills Training: A Manual of Guidelines*. Chichester: John Wiley and Sons.

Perkins, E.R. (1979) *Parentcraft: A Comparative Study of Teaching Method*. Leverhulme Health Education Project Occasional Papers No. 16. Nottingham: University of Nottingham.

Perkins, E.R. and Craig, E. (1981) *Parentcraft Teaching, the Basic Skills*. Paper for limited circulation, Health Education Council.

Perkins, E.R. and Morris, B. (1979) *Preparation for Parenthood: a Critique of the Concept*. Leverhulme Health Education Project Occasional Papers No. 17. Nottingham: University of Nottingham.

Reynolds, W. and Cormack, D.F.S. (1985) Clinical teaching of group dynamics and evaluation of a trial clinical teaching programme. *Nurse Education Today*, **5**: 101–108.

Roberts, H., Wotten, I.D.P., Kane, K.M. and Harnett, W.E. (1953) The value of antenatal preparation. *Journal of Obstetrics and Gynaecology of the British Empire*. **60**: 404–408.

Royal College of Midwives (1966) *Preparation for Parenthood*. London: RCM.

Royal College of Midwives Scottish Board (1986) *Annual Report*. Edinburgh: RCM.

Royal College of Nursing (1983) *Thinking about Health Visiting*. Discussion paper produced by the RCN Health Visitors Advisory Group. London: RCN.

Sweet, B. (1984) Midwives in clinical practice. *Nursing Times*, **80**(23): 60–62.

Taylor, A. (1985) Antenatal classes and the consumer: mother and father views. *Health Education Journal*, **44**: 79–82.

Vehvilainen, K. (1984) *Interaction, Labour, Midwife, Mother*. Paper presented to WENR/RCN Research Society Conference, London.

Wagner, A.C. (1973) Changing teaching behaviour: a comparison of micro teaching and cognitive discrimination training. *Journal of Educational Psychology*, **64**: 299–305.

9

IMPLICATIONS FOR PRACTICE

Penny Jones

In the long history of midwifery, research is still in its relative infancy. As a student midwife in 1977 undertaking the, as it was then, 12-month training course, the subject did not form part of the curriculum, and on receiving the letter informing me that I had passed the final exams and could now call myself a midwife, I remember heaving a sigh of relief and cheerfully thinking, 'I'll never have to look at another textbook again', which just goes to show how wrong one can be, because of course, midwifery is like most things in that it is constantly changing.

It is rather naive to believe that since babies continue to be conceived and born in much the same way as they always have been, the skills and knowledge gained during training are still applicable, no matter how long the midwife has been in practice. Even if one were to read no more than the popular press, it would soon become apparent that that belief is quite erroneous. Midwifery is a rapidly altering health-care field, affected by technological, social and scientific changes – and midwives must change too. Whereas perinatal and maternal mortality rates have fallen, consumer dissatisfaction is rising. Increased obstetric intervention is a cause of concern for many midwives, and as the clientele become more aware of their rights and want more participation in their care, midwives are forced to become more litigation conscious. There is also growing pressure to provide a more cost-effective service.

Beleagured on all sides, the midwife of today must be a more accountable professional if she is to retain her credibility. One means by which the midwife can do this is by constantly updating her skills and knowledge (Sweet, 1986) and although there are 5-yearly refresher courses to attend, the midwife cannot rely on these to do it all for her. Nor is it reasonable to expect a 1-week course to fulfil the responsibility to 'take every reasonable opportunity to maintain and improve professional knowledge and experience' (UKCC, 1986). However, reading relevant journals and research reports goes a long way towards doing so.

Most of my own knowledge of research was gained through the Advanced Diploma in Midwifery course, although by the time I undertook this I had learned a little more than I knew when just qualified and had already witnessed a change in midwifery practice, brought about by research. Routine perineal shaving was abandoned, largely because of Romney's (1980) research, and the use of enemas prior to delivery was more selective (Romney and Gordon, 1981). All concerned seem to appreciate the change – the mothers especially because they now had an element of choice, whereas previously the enema seemed to have been accepted as a dreaded but necessary part of the birth process.

It is not to be expected that the findings of all research directed at midwifery will be as simple to implement as the above examples or that midwives will find them as easily acceptable. The very nature of research is to question, or critically evaluate, and in doing so to challenge beliefs and/or practices held almost sacred over a number of years, some of which are far harder than others to shake. When a midwife believes that shaving a perineum or giving an enema prior to delivery facilitates events, she will do so, distasteful as it may be. When she actually knows that it is of little or no benefit as a routine procedure, it is easy for her to restrict these procedures to cases where there is a genuine necessity. It is far harder to dispense with long-cherished beliefs about, for example, breast feeding. This is self-evident to any midwife working on a postnatal ward, faced with yet more distressed mothers upset by conflicting advice on the subject.

Midwifery has some long-acknowledged problem areas, which many midwives would like to see resolved. Unfortunately, research does not provide instant answers and should not be expected to, but what it can do is give some insight into the nature and extent of a problem. This may eventually lead to a solution or, alternatively, promote further research. Some of those topics that most concern the practising midwife of today are the subjects of the research chapters of this book.

The midwife is responsible for giving 'the necessary supervision, care and advice to women during pregnancy, labour and the postpartum period' (UKCC, 1986), and one of the implications to be drawn from Chapters 2–8 above is that this could be done more effectively. Another is that the education of midwives – and, with regard to their role in maternity care, of health visitors – needs some re-appraisal. It also seems that not enough midwives fully appreciate the need for research and its importance to our profession. It is further implied, by a lack of willingness to participate in the research process, that not enough of those involved in maternity care are willing to be seen to question what we do and why we do it.

Antenatal care, 'the perfect example of preventive medicine' (House of Commons, 1980), has long suffered from criticism, and it is therefore appropriate that it should be the subject of two of the studies presented. As long ago as 50 years there were complaints being made about lack of continuity of care, although few of the early authors recognised that consumer doubt about efficacy of care, long waiting periods and difficulties in attending, particularly if they had other children, might be the cause of this (Oakley, 1982). This was long before the Peel Report of 1970 and the Short Report of 1980, and the hospitalisation recommended led to antenatal clinics being centralised at the hospital where confinement was to take place. The continuity of care that should have resulted from this did not, in fact, materialise. Oakley (1979), in a study of first time mothers, found that women were still complaining of feeling depersonalised, 'like items on a conveyor belt or assembly line'. They felt that there was a lack of continuity of care, some being seen by as many as nine different doctors, and two-thirds had never before seen the person who delivered their baby.

What did result from hospitalisation, however, was a steady decline of the community midwifery service. The study on which Davies and Evans (Chapter 7) report has sought to redress the balance and give more support to the mothers who most need it, both of which it seems to have achieved. In several respects, this project resembles that of Boddy et al (1981), whose antenatal care scheme at Sighthill in Edinburgh has proved very successful, both in terms of providing continuity of care and of restoring job satisfaction to the primary health-care members involved. The trust these community midwives have gained from their clientele is something that many midwives would surely like to achieve since it obviously facilitates so much. It is to be hoped that the completed analysis leads to its establishment on a permanent basis, and that other midwives and health authorities will consider implementing similar schemes. This project also serves to demonstrate that what was thought to be an inefficient method of care actually works far better for all concerned than does the method that replaced it. Community midwifery care has so much more to offer in terms of making the birth of a baby a 'normal' event than is perhaps recognised by midwifery staff and doctors used to little other than hospital-based maternity care. There is growing concern among the midwife's clientele about the over-medicalisation of childbirth, and projects like this could do much to restore it to a more normal perspective.

Antenatal education is an important aspect of maternity care but nevertheless it still suffers from the problems common to antenatal care in general. In her description of the antenatal classes of the Newcastle project, Davies says that the mothers did not want to be 'taught' but they wanted to learn. It is quite possible that a great many other mothers feel the same way. In view of the many criticisms that have been levelled at antenatal education and the need for these classes to continue, it is time we took a realistic look at the manner of teaching pregnant women. Indeed, these classes have been described as being as much interventions as are some other aspects of modern antenatal care (Enkin, 1982), so there is much room for improvement.

As Murphy-Black and Faulkner (Chapter 8) point out in the introduction to their study, communication skills are not really as strong as could be wished among nurses and those involved in maternity care, and more education is needed in teaching skills. In the past antenatal educators have always 'taught' rather than facilitated learning, so it is interesting to see what can be achieved by applying a different method of teaching to the educators themselves. The self-selected group derived far more benefit from the teaching and group skills training course (even though the improvement was less than in other studies) than did the manager-selected groups. Some would say that this is only to be expected given human nature, but the self-selected group emerged as having become better facilitators of learning, despite the two groups being evenly matched for previous teaching experience, than did the manager-selected group, who only seemed to have got better at filling silences. As the authors conclude, unless antenatal educators themselves become aware of their developmental needs, little will change. Here is an underlying message for all midwives, that the desire for change must come from oneself, not from outside. Some insight is provided into the future for education, but how much credence will be given to this study by those most nearly concerned remains to be seen.

There can be no doubt that labour is painful but midwives have probably all noticed that there can be a marked variation from one labouring mother to another. In studying labour pain Niven confirms this but has also come up with some other interesting findings. It is pleasing to discover that what is described as a 'rule of thumb', used by many midwives in trying to assess how much pain multigravidae may be expected to experience, is valid. However, there is more to Niven's findings than just this. Nowdays it is standard practice to discuss pain relief in labour with primigravid women on their admission to the labour ward, and it is usual to enquire of multigravid women what analgesia, if any, was used last time and how effective it was. Niven's study suggests that it might also be of value to know a woman's previous history of pain experience, on the basis that this can have an effect on how labour pain is experienced. But it also poses the question of how best to apply Niven's findings –if midwives are to employ a more holistic approach to maternity care, perhaps they should be re-evaluating both how they treat the whole subject of pain in labour throughout the antenatal period and how they see it themselves.

To do or not to do – this is the question faced by midwives in their dealings with labouring women when it comes to deciding whether or not an episiotomy is necessary. This has to be one of the most controversial issues midwives have to contend with in daily practice. The changes brought about by the increased technology now associated with labour can perhaps be blamed for forcing the scissor hand of many a midwife, but the current episiotomy rate is nonetheless alarming. Sleep's research (Chapter 2) points out that all midwives must evaluate their rationale for performing this procedure, since she is able to show us that there is no sound evidence that it is of benefit to either the mother or her baby. Midwives are in a particularly vulnerable position over performing an episiotomy – the mother of today is in general better informed than in the past and some are now categorically stating that they do not want an episiotomy. To do so against a mother's expressed wishes could constitute an assault for which midwives may be liable and, in fact, this study shows that there are no real grounds for the present high number of episiotomies being performed. While midwives may not want to be responsible for severe perineal trauma, it is also very clear that an episiotomy may not be the best means of preventing this from occurring.

Normal delivery is the province of the midwife, and as her role extends to include perineal repair, she has a greater responsibility than ever before for the future quality of life of her clientele. In order to give the best possible standard of care it must be ensured that practice is based on knowledge rather than on tradition. It is also apparent that more consideration should be given to adequate analgesia for episiotomy, perineal repair and perineal pain in the puerperium. Nor can midwives afford to forget about the complications of stress incontinence and dyspareunia, from which a significant percentage of women may suffer following a normal delivery.

Infant feeding is currently the subject of a positive wealth of literature and, in theory, it should be the success story of the decade. This is far from being the case, however, and there are still too many mothers who are left feeling a failure because, despite a firm belief in the value of breast feeding, many of them give up. The most common time for this is around 6 weeks, with one or more reasons being given for discontinuing. Wright (Chapter 4) examines the highly complex issue of infant feeding from a psychological perspective, providing a fascinating look at the behavioural pattern of babies in this respect, the changes that occur and how their mothers perceive this behaviour.

It has previously been shown in a study by Houston et al (1983) that for 66% of mothers their baby's behaviour did not improve following the change from breast to bottle, so not all difficulties are resolved simply by giving up breast feeding. Could it be that we just do not have enough understanding of infant behaviour? Wright's study illustrates that this may be so. He finds that babies behave in a particular manner, with a clear difference between the sexes, and that their mothers do not always correctly interpret this behaviour. Most marked changes occur at 5–7 weeks of age, which is when as many as half of mothers stop breast feeding. There is a tendency to look at feeding problems from a physical and maternal viewpoint, not giving the baby much consideration at all. It seems that if mothers could be given a better understanding of their baby's behaviour, more of them might succeed in 'overcoming the 6-week hurdle'. In the last 10 years, there have been many improvements in our knowledge of infant feeding. More mothers now want to breast feed and more – but not enough – are successful. Wright concludes that mothers should be better prepared to deal with the problems and realities associated with breast feeding, recommending that we teach mothers to anticipate them while reinforcing the information that they already have.

Holden (Chapter 5) highlights the lack of knowledge and awareness of postnatal depression (PND) that prevails among both parents and health-care professionals. In her study mothers were identified as suffering from PND using a self-report scale specifically designed for this purpose, and a study group received counselling from health visitors who had been prepared for this role. This study group showed a significantly higher recovery rate than did the control mothers and, in addition, these mothers developed a good relationship with their health visitors and a better understanding of her role. All parents felt they should have known more about PND.

Both this study and that of Wright imply that maternity care as it stands at present is not meeting the needs of parents. During both the antenatal and postnatal periods, midwives are failing to educate parents adequately about the realities of their new role, the difficulties they may encounter and what to do about them should they arise.

Bryar (Chapter 6) describes the implementation of a change in practice. Recognition of the fragmented nature of maternity care led to the development of a midwifery assessment and the use of the nursing process in an attempt to provide continuity of care. Once fully implemented the effect of this change was evaluated to see whether or not using the nursing process had brought about more individualised care of clients. Staff were given a questionnaire to complete so that the researcher could evaluate their views and knowledge of the nursing process. Unfortunately, there was only a 30% response rate to the questionnaire; therefore the findings of this part of her study cannot be taken as truly predictive on a broader scale. Observation of staff showed care to be still largely standardised and routine based rather than individualised, and the nursing process was found to be underutilised, although this appears to be partly due to restrictive hospital policies. While this study demonstrates some of the problems that can be encountered in undertaking research, it is particularly interesting and calls for more research in this area. It is also very encouraging that staff in the study hospital have continued with the process of change.

In conclusion, these research chapters offer new avenues for exploration of maternity care. Midwives and health visitors are presented with an opportunity to take their findings and use them to improve practice or to ignore them, rendering the profession the poorer by so doing. The principal function of research is to 'look again' at aspects of our everyday work, and it would not be realistic to expect the questions that it asks always to come up with conclusions that are particularly palatable. Research cannot be ignored because its findings are disliked, nor is it possible to ignore some pieces of work and accept others simply because they happen to vindicate personal beliefs. All research that is relevant to practice should be considered. Those involved in maternity care need to take more of an interest in research and gain a fuller understanding of what it is, how it works and its potential, for it has a great deal to offer the profession. This is the major implication of this book.

What research can give is the stimulus to bring about change and provide a better, more effective service. It can help midwives to meet more of the clients' needs more of the time, and give added enthusiasm for what is done as well as a more stimulating atmosphere in which to do it. And perhaps most of all, it can offer a future in which there are still midwives in the role of practitioners. By becoming a research-based profession, midwives could have the means to ensure the future of midwifery rather than allowing their role to be eroded until they are reduced to being mere obstetric nurses.

One thing is certain – there is much about current maternity care that could be better and the responsibility to bring about the necessary change to achieve this end lies with the maternity care workers of today. The researchers in this book have shown the initiative by asking questions and it is therefore up to midwives to respond by evaluating and updating their practice. Doing everything in the same way as it has always been done, and never looking at textbooks again once qualified, is undemanding but inevitably tedious when there are so many interesting new possibilities. Research offers us an exciting challenge – are we equal to that challenge? I hope that we are.

REFERENCES

Boddy, K., Parboosingh, I.J.T. and Shepherd, W.C. (1981) *A Schematic Approach to Prenatal Care*. Unpublished document available from Dr K. Boddy, Dept. of Obstetrics and Gynaecology, Edinburgh University.

Enkin, M. (1982) In: *Effectiveness and Satisfaction in Ante-Natal Care*, Enkin, M. and Chalmers, I. (eds.) pp. 151–161. Lavenham: Spastics International Medical Publications.

House of Commons (1980) *Second Report of the Social Services Committee on Perinatal and Neonatal Mortality* (Chairman: Short). London: HMSO.

Houston, M., Howie, P. and McNeilly, A. (1983) Midwifery forum 2: Breast-feeding. *Nursing Mirror*, 156(6).

Oakley, A. (1979) *From Here to Maternity*. Harmondsworth: Penguin.

Oakley, A. (1982) In: *Effectiveness and Satisfaction in Ante-Natal Care*, Enkin, M. and Chalmers, I. (eds.) pp. 1–19. Lavenham: Spastics International Medical Publications.

Romney, M.L. (1980) Pre-delivery shaving: an unjustified assault? *Journal of Obstetrics and Gynaecology*, 1(1): 33–35.

Romney, M.L. and Gordon, J. (1981) Is your enema really necessary? *British Medical Journal*, 1269–1271.

Sweet, B.R. (1986) 'From the first day of the rest of your career' . . . Continuing education of the midwife. *Midwives Chronicle*, **99**(1): vii–ix.

United Kingdom Central Council for Nursing, Midwifery and Health Visiting (1986) *A Midwife's Code of Practice*, 1st edn. London: UKCC.

10

IMPLICATIONS FOR MANAGEMENT

Glynis Mayes

Writing in 1977, Jean Walker noted that the need to develop and apply scientific knowledge of the management of normal childbirth had not gained acceptance by professionals in the maternity services. In this chapter an attempt will be made to assess whether or not this can be considered a true reflection of the situation today and to identify the responsibilities that fall to managers and teachers in this respect.

The decline in perinatal and maternal mortality rates throughout this century demonstrates that childbirth has become far safer for both mother and baby. A variety of factors is likely to have contributed to this very real achievement, including improvement in standards of general health and living conditions and also developments in medical science. Midwives have played their part by developing high levels of skill and expertise in operating and interpreting the outputs of this technology, which then assists the obstetrician in making a diagnosis and prescribing a course of treatment or management. Midwifery, however, encompasses a wider field, which extends beyond the parameters of medical prescription to include the provision of emotional support and preparation for childbirth and parenthood. Besides technical and practical competence, midwifery demands a deep understanding of the experiences that the mother and her family undergo. It involves recognising fears and needs, giving encouragement and promoting confidence for independence and participating in decision-making. A glance at the contents of this book illustrates a range of midwifery issues that lie outside the scope of the obstetrician.

Houston and Weatherston (1986) point out that midwifery is unique in that midwives have a perspective of childbearing that is different from the obstetrician, viewing the process as essentially normal, with intervention applied as necessary in emergency situations. The midwife's role allows her to work closely with women throughout their childbearing so that she is able to become aware of the expectations and unmet needs of mothers and their families, and this poses questions about current practice beyond the consideration of physical safety alone. These questions give rise to yet more and, as the answers are not to be found in medical texts, midwives must look for the answers themselves. In this search midwives can add to the body of knowledge on the processes of pregnancy, childbirth and parenthood and can develop a greater personal understanding of the range of needs and the ways in which midwives can contribute to meeting those needs. The accumulation of evidence and data provides a basis for midwives to demonstrate the justification for their true role.

CONSUMERISM

The trend, begun in the 1950s, towards hospital confinements and the increased medicalisation of childbirth to achieve a 'safe delivery' concentrates on the physical aspects of care based on the diagnosis and treatment of the abnormal and pathological. It should not be forgotten, though, that maternal and perinatal mortality rates had already begun to fall significantly before this move into the hospital. Walker (1977) draws attention to the view that the medical model of curing illness by diagnosis and treatment may not always be appropriate as a framework for health care and can even produce undesirable side-effects, as in the process of turning healthy childbearing women into patients for treatment in hospitals.

Sir Graham Godber, as Chief Medical Officer, pointed out (Department of Health and Social Security, 1968) that the advances in obstetric knowledge had been successful in lowering mortality figures in childbirth and that the time might have come for more consideration of the qualitative aspects of childbirth. This has since been endorsed by the Short Report (House of Commons, 1980) and the Maternity Care in Action Reports of the Maternity Services Advisory Committee (1982, 1984, 1985). Cartwright (1979) maintains that midwives have a vital role to play in the development of a service in which mothers play a more dominant and less subservient role. This notion has been promoted by consumers, as in their response to the BBC 'That's Life' programme's probe into maternity care, and also by pressure groups such as the National Childbirth Trust challenging professions on the effects of the belief that no birth can be considered normal except in retrospect.

There are numerous accounts of dissatisfaction resulting from intervention in labour that have been attributed to long-term problems such as postnatal depression and difficulties in bonding. Anxiety and intimidation have been reported as the consequence of attending crowded antenatal clinics, where, because all women are required to see a doctor, the medical staff are too overworked to allow more than a cursory few minutes with each one. The negative aspects of this system can be seen to counteract any benefits derived from the clinic visit, and the stirring accounts of the distress and frustration felt by the women, together with the enormous waste of midwifery skills revealed in the Chelsea College Nursing Education Research Unit midwifery project (Robinson et al, 1983), are clear pointers to managers for re-organising the provision of antenatal care. The widespread development of midwives' clinics is evidence of a response to these findings and there are more radical innovations in which women are booked with teams of midwives who are able to give continuity of care on a more personal basis, or where antenatal care is predominantly community based.

At a time when quality of care and consumerism feature prominently in the current style of management (DHSS, 1983), initiating and acting on consumer research takes on a vital importance for managers. The maternity services often occupy a high profile in the local community and it is an area in which the provision of care must be particularly responsive to local demands, requiring the planners and professionals to be closely 'in tune' with the characteristics of the community and to be sensitive to any changes in those characteristics. Managers are, therefore, required to evaluate the forms of care offered, identify needs and problems, measure the effectiveness of the service in meeting those needs and set objectives for the service on the basis of that information. Meeting those objectives can be a demanding challenge, especially if a marked change in approach or practice is indicated, and this is where firm evidence, and not merely opinion or political pressure, is essential.

STANDARDS OF PRACTICE

Establishing and setting standards is another feature of the current management philosophy, and many midwifery managers also carry the statutory responsibility for ensuring that all midwifery practice fulfils the requirements of the Nurses, Midwives and Health Visitors Act as set out in the Midwives Rules and the Code of Practice (UKCC, 1986). The code, which lays down the principles on which professional practice is based, states in the introduction:

> 'Each midwife as a practitioner of midwifery is accountable for her own practice in whatever environment she practises. The standard of practice in the delivery of midwifery care shall be that which is acceptable in the context of current knowledge and clinical developments.'

The code then goes on to outline the definition of the midwife and the activities encompassed within that role. No longer, however, are the actual duties prescribed, so the responsibility falls to each individual midwife to make her own judgments about the most appropriate care to meet the needs of the mother and baby. It is incumbent on managers and teachers to ensure that midwives are equipped with the knowledge for and skill in decision-making to enable them not only to deliver that care effectively but also to justify, in a logical way, the reasoning behind a particular course of action. That knowledge needs to be grounded on firm evidence not merely on accepted dogma and should be sufficiently broad to cover familiarity with a range of possible practices and theories. Throughout training the relevant research findings should be introduced to substantiate the theory and practice when they are programmed into the course.

Local policies should allow and encourage midwives to respond more sensitively to patients' needs, by departing from the general routines when circumstances indicate that it would be appropriate.

Bryar's study (Chapter 6) of the introduction of a process of individualised care gives examples of care that did not respond to mothers' needs but followed the accepted routine instead. Perhaps this indicates a lack of confidence in the practitioners to risk stepping out of line or embarking on a course of action that may have further implications. In order to instil confidence in mothers the midwife needs to feel secure in her own judgments and actions, so managers have a responsibility in the development of their staff to encourage midwives to draw on a range of knowledge to build up their expertise. The results of research provide an important source of this knowledge.

STUDIES OF THE PROCESS OF CHILDBEARING

Scientific observation of physiological processes adds to the body of knowledge that forms the basis for planning care. It increases understanding of the mother's perspective, creating a greater awareness of her feelings and requirements, and improves the effectiveness of the care provided.

The perception of pain is confined to the one individual; it cannot be shared and, as such, can be a very isolating experience. Pain is clearly a very important aspect of labour and there is a wide range of attitudes relating to this type of pain. The terms 'low pain threshold' and 'high pain threshold' carry judgmental overtones, and the debate in favour of and against epidural anaesthesia involves views about whether pain is, in itself, a vital part of the birth experience. There are value judgments surrounding notions of conquering pain or giving in, with insinuations of failure and weakness. The mother may feel anger, directed towards the baby, because of the pain that has to be endured. Midwives are not immune to these attitudes, which may unconsciously affect their practice. Many midwives display a strong desire for the mother to be as comfortable as possible and find it disturbing if she is in obvious pain. Because of this wish to relieve the suffering they may find themselves accused of forcing analgesia on labouring women.

Niven's study (Chapter 3) on pain in labour provides important information on the intensity of pain, analysing a subjective experience in a way that allows for comparison with pain in other labours or with different causes of pain. The results confirm the severity of pain in labour and the diagram comparing labour pain with other types of pain places this experience in context. The range in the scores indicates that caution is necessary when making predictions, but the evidence that previous experience of pain is related to the intensity of labour pain adds to our understanding of how individuals deal with pain. This awareness makes it possible to improve the quality of joint decisions made by the mother, midwife and doctor in the management of the labour and pain relief.

Helping women to prepare for labour requires sensitivity if the help is to be effective. In maintaining credibility the information offered must be realistic when the question of pain is tackled. Midwives face a dilemma that, recognising the need for realism, there is a risk of creating such fear and anxiety that the thought of labour becomes a nightmare and any joy in the actual birth is lost. Experienced midwives handle this in a number of ways, giving an explanation of the help available to alleviate the pain to ensure that the mother remains in control. Knowledge of the results of this study may be helpful to the midwife when discussing pain in labour at antenatal classes, when taking an antenatal history and when supporting a woman in her labour.

The second study that enhances our understanding of a normal process is the work on early feeding behaviour. A wealth of research has revealed the high inci-dence of mothers giving up breast feeding within the first few weeks and Wright

(Chapter 4) relates this to his observation of the feeding patterns of the baby. Breast feeding is an activity controlled by the mother and she is influenced by a number of factors, including her perception of her baby's need for food and her assessment of the level of satisfaction that it gives. Wright's demonstration of the inaccuracy of the mothers' estimations of their babies' hunger is surprising and indicates a divergence between the babies' actual needs and the mothers' recognition of those needs. He suggests that the critical point that determines the continuation of breast feeding coincides with the period at 5–7 weeks old when the baby's pattern of food intake changes. This suggests that the mother misinterprets the changing demands of the baby so that when the baby is not satisfied this is attributed to inadequate lactation. It remains to be tested whether or not an improvement in the mother's knowledge would affect the success of breast feeding. This would require the midwife and health visitor to work closely together, beginning with the antenatal preparation to 'provide a more accurate picture of what breast feeding entails to prevent unrealistic expectations', a need highlighted by a number of mothers in the study.

There are heavy demands on a mother during those first 6 weeks when she has to contend with lack of sleep and hormonal changes. Numerous studies have recommended the need for help and support with feeding during this time. The findings of this particular study may point to the benefit of helping the mother to recognise the signals from her baby and of reinforcing the knowledge gained antenatally. Consistency in approach by the midwife and health visitor is important and this is enhanced if there is continuity in the advice through good hand out of information. Another interesting finding from this work is the failure of some bottle feeding mothers to recognise that their babies' hunger is satisfied. As the author points out, this is likely to result in overfeeding and suggests the need for professionals to give help and information with this.

EVALUATIVE STUDY OF A MIDWIFERY PRACTICE

Many procedures in midwifery are rooted in tradition; some gain almost universal acceptance while others attract support in opposing camps. Perineal shaving had become so entrenched in routine preparation for labour that the work of Romney (1980), demonstrating that shaving had no effect on infection, was received with some surprise. Episiotomy has attracted forceful opinions from pressure groups and professionals, so it is fitting that this particular study was undertaken by a midwife. Sleep's paper (Chapter 2) includes a useful consideration of the ethical issues, which feature to some extent in all research but particularly in a randomised controlled trial such as this, where there are widely held views on the indications for the procedure and where there is a risk of harm associated with either course of management.

The conclusions derived from the study indicate that there is no evidence for the commonly held beliefs on the healing of episiotomies as compared with tears or the degree of trauma that may be incurred. Since 10% of the mothers from the group where episiotomy was restricted sustained no trauma at all, the justification for this invasive procedure is called into question.

The results of this study should be incorporated in midwifery teaching when preparing midwives for the decisions and judgments they will be faced with in the course of their practice and the context in which the procedure should be regarded. To reinforce that approach it is essential that the practising midwives are aware of recent findings when supervising learners, demonstrating that the quality of practice is enhanced by new knowledge. It will be interesting to note the degree to which the results of this study will influence midwifery practice or whether midwives will justify their judgment and actions by their own belief.

Regular evaluation and review of practice is fundamental to professionalism and professional accountability, and managers and teachers of midwifery should aim to create an environment and culture that is receptive to questioning current values and policies and which encourages innovation.

A SEARCH FOR AN ANSWER TO A PROBLEM

Another form of research is to identify a problem and to look for a solution that can be evaluated. This is the approach followed in the study Holden describes on the detection and management of postnatal depression by health visitors (Chapter 5).

Although there is growing awareness of the scale of postnatal depression, studies have shown that the number actually treated remains low. The nature of the condition differs from other forms of psychiatric disorders and, possibly because there is a spontaneous recovery, its management has received little attention from professionals. This undermines the misery and bewilderment experienced by the mothers and the drastic impact and long-term implications on the family. This study looks at whether or not the problem can be addressed effectively through the existing services and evaluates means by which this could be achieved. The development of the Edinburgh Postnatal Depression Scale not only shows that it is an effective method of identifying mothers who are in need of help but also throws light on the issue that it is not easily recognised by professionals in the services as they are currently delivered. It is moving to learn that the mothers found that completing the depression scale was therapeutic in itself as they felt that it gave them permission to express their feelings. It is also worth noting that the image the mothers had of the health visitor's role prevented them from raising the subject spontaneously, whereas participation in the study changed their perception of her approachability and her job. Perhaps midwives could be more positive in this respect when preparing the mother for transfer to the health visitor.

The value of counselling is being demonstrated for a growing range of situations, and this study shows that it was particularly effective in contributing to the recovery of mothers from postnatal depression. Attention is drawn to the fact that both the mothers and the fathers in the study stressed the importance of antenatal education in that, had they known more about postnatal depression, they would have had the courage to seek help more readily. This indicates the need for midwives to gain more knowledge on the subject in order to introduce discussion of postnatal depression with the mothers antenatally, which would include consideration of recognising early signs and the benefit of seeking help.

The limitations of the effectiveness of antenatal education constitute a problem that was addressed by setting up a training course in teaching and groupwork skills. The evaluation of the course, undertaken by Murphy-Black and Faulkner (Chapter 8) involved a questionnaire study as well as observation both before and after attendance at the training course. The observation entailed interaction analysis, a check-list of environmental and physical aspects and a description of the behaviour of the class members.

Communication is of fundamental importance in midwifery. Since the mother is in control of her life-style and actions, all care and advice is only effective to the extent to which the mother chooses to accept it. This applies to all midwifery care but is particularly applicable to antenatal education. The manner in which information is introduced and put over is crucial to the receptivity of the mothers attending classes and the use they make of that information.

It was noted that the levels of interaction between teachers and mothers was generally low and it would be interesting to know something of the mothers' expectations. Did they see the class as a source of information, having discussed their personal worries or fears with the midwife at the antenatal clinic, or would they have liked more full, in-depth discussion in the class but felt inhibited or lacked the opportunity?

Although 'providing a programme of parenthood preparation and a complete preparation for childbirth' is listed in the activities of a midwife in the Midwife's Code of Practice (UKCC, 1986), it is a duty that does not appeal readily to every midwife. Confidence is gained through specific training but communication skills should feature as a vital component of midwifery training throughout the entire course. Incorporated within this should be a more thorough preparation of teaching and groupwork skills as necessary tools for midwifery practice.

The differences observed between the self-selected and manager-selected course participants are of particular interest. The value of helping staff to become aware of their own need for development can be seen in their responsiveness to further training and the benefits derived from it. This has implications not only for developing staff to give a better service but also for the individuals to fulfil their professional accountability.

TRIAL AND EVALUATION OF NEW FORMS OF CARE

It could be said that research generates further research, in which studies of a subject may develop into a multistage enquiry. For example, a local audit may reveal a high incidence of postpartum haemorrhage when compared with national figures. This may lead to an investigation and comparison of methods employed in the management of the third stage of labour. In such a study, Moore and Levy (1981) showed that the blood loss was less if the signs of separation of the placenta were awaited prior to applying controlled cord traction. These findings may cause a unit to decide to alter its policy, and in order to test the effectiveness of the new regime, a third generation study may be set up.

The innovation may be relatively simple, such as testing a different design of mucus extractor or changing the methods used in treatment of the umbilical cord. A highly complex new scheme of total care may be introduced, such as the 'know your midwife scheme' in Tooting, London, where a team of midwives books and carries out complete care for low-risk mothers. The study of the implementation of the midwifery process by Bryar (Chapter 6) falls into this last category. Because there were a number of aspects to this project, including the development of appropriate documentation and patient allocation within the antenatal clinic and wards in order to achieve individualised care, the planning and implementation formed part of the study. This involved consideration of the process of change within an organisation, in this case beginning with in-service training programmes, developing and piloting assessment and care plans and introducing systems to give better continuity of care. This was supported by regular meetings and by a co-ordinating group of nursing officers and tutors. A cross-sectional study was then undertaken to assess the extent to which individualised care had been achieved and to examine the views of the staff; this included the use of non-participant observation, questionnaires, interviews and analysis of records.

This list of activities gives some idea of the enormity of the task of introducing such a fundamental change, drawing attention to the importance of ongoing education and full consultation as preparation for the staff, developing and planning the new systems and the actual implementation, involving full participation of the staff involved. Despite the thoroughness of the ground work, the cross-sectional study revealed examples of standardised care in all areas, in some cases determined by hospital policies. Analysis of the records showed a lack of identification of individual problems and there was a disparity between the large number of problems and care provided and the absence or vagueness of recording problems and plans. This showed that, at the time of the study, care was still routinised, fragmented and unresponsive to individual needs, in spite of the fact that the staff had indicated that they valued individualised care.

The author points out that change is a gradual process and suggests that consideration of the intra- and extra-organisational constraints may have contributed to greater change than would an educational programme. Possibly, the changes proposed were too far removed from the framework of the existing model of care, so that more attention should be directed to the underlying beliefs and values that comprise the ideology of the particular cultural setting. It is noted that the process of change begun in the project is continuing, which may indicate that a change in behaviour can lead to a change in beliefs even if the change in behaviour is imposed.

The community midwifery project is another example of introducing and evaluating the effects of a different form of care, this time by providing a more intensive input of midwifery care in women's own homes.

While the full results of the study are not yet available, the benefits of neighbourhood midwifery support for women in socially deprived conditions are discussed. Because of the vulnerability of the mothers, continuity of care is seen to be particularly important and proved to be rewarding for the midwives. It is suggested, therefore, that the individualised care and support that a community midwife can offer in the home is more appropriate in these circumstances than is a system that requires women to conform to the hospital regime. The author indicates that the study will also include an analysis of the work of the midwives, which could be valuable information to add to the work on the role of the midwife by the Chelsea College midwifery project and the National Perinatal Epidemiological Unit in Oxford.

RESEARCH AS AN AGENT FOR CHANGE

Implementing the results of research can be difficult and time-consuming. Often the findings do not offer a definitive answer but may be applied in a number of ways, or similar studies may even lead to contradictory conclusions. This leaves the midwife to make a choice, from a number of options, of which evidence to accept and act on. Skill is needed in examining the methodology of research projects and, in particular, in questioning the justification for the conclusion reached. Therefore, there has to be some means of familiarising midwives with research concepts and terminology as well as with the details of methods, techniques and analysis. This should feature not only in basic midwifery training but also in ongoing education, although not neces- sarily as a subject in isolation. Research is more meaningful if incorporated in the teaching of midwifery practice where the evidence is drawn from pieces of research. This is particularly important if midwives are to learn about the application of research to practice and to recognise that it makes a positive contribution to the care that is given. Post-basic education through which midwives can learn about re- search includes research appreciation refresher courses and English National Board Course 995 in research, and the subject is included in the Advanced Diploma of Midwifery. The aim is to introduce midwives to research skills, to help them to become more receptive to the implications and findings of research and to point them towards constantly reviewing and questioning practices in the light of ac- cumulating knowledge.

Bond (1981) urges midwives to 'ask repeatedly, what is the knowledge base for our practices? Are they in step with the current state of knowledge or are they merely rituals?' Experience is probably the chief way by which midwives develop their expertise but experiences are constrained by the situations of the working environment and the knowledge fed in. There is a growing number of published studies that lead midwives to question the relevance of routine procedures including perineal shaving and the administration of enemas (Romney, 1980; Romney and Gordon, 1981), episiotomies, cord care, controlled cord traction (Moore and Levy, 1981), postnatal care (Ball, 1983) and antenatal history taking (Methven, 1982). It is not enough, however, to know about it; the findings must be used and converted into action if care is to be improved and the profession is to grow.

Hofer (1975) questioned whether or not medical and nursing policies, hospital design and obstetric and paediatric procedures should be altered substantially on the basis of research evidence. He cautioned against making radical changes in the light of research misinterpreted and exploited by pressure groups. Discipline is called for when reading research reports, and careful evaluation of the effects of changes is necessary to see whether or not they achieve what is required. Boyd and Sellars' study (1982) indicates that many mothers prefer babies to be taken to the nursery at night but to remain with them during the day. Ball (1985) describes how her work confirmed this, so she referred to the text of Klaus and Kennell (1976), often quoted as advocating 24-hour rooming-in. She found that they never recommended this at all, but favoured complete access by mother and baby during the day, with the baby brought to her for feeding at night.

Introducing change can be threatening as established patterns of practice are overturned. This anxiety can be reduced if staff are actively involved in demonstrating the need for change. Houston and Weatherston (1986) have described the value of setting up practice-based research groups to provide a resource for midwives wishing to improve their knowledge of research and methods and to promote awareness of the importance of research-based practice. Two such groups were studied and were shown to improve practice, to generate confidence and self-esteem, to improve communication and mutual respect among colleagues and to create a vehicle for change and development.

Ottoway (1979), writing about change agents in the workplace, has suggested that everyone is a change agent to some degree in some part of his or her life. He identifies change generators, who have the insight and energy to question and create change, change implementors, who, when they learn of the need, move rapidly to creating change in their environment, and change adopters, who, when change seems inevitable, integrate it into their practice. There are also change resisters, who, in some ways, provide a system of checks and balances to prevent constant change destabilising the system.

In an environment in which research is taking place the participation of the midwives can motivate their commitment to acting on the results. Facilitating the research of others, however, by becoming involved in collecting or contributing data can also have negative effects. This arises when the purpose is unclear and when contributors do not receive any feedback despite devoting time and energy to collecting information. Managers play an important role in determining the conditions for this type of exercise and in making sure that the findings are made available. Managers can also be effective in motivating staff to see the relevance of studies and in gaining their co-operation. New ideas will be accepted more readily if they are consistent with the beliefs and approach to the existing framework of provision of care. If the proposed change represents a marked departure from those beliefs, attention needs to be focused on addressing the belief system to determine a new ideology from which the proposed change can be seen to develop. Power systems, communication systems and support warrant consideration beforehand to ensure that they facilitate the change rather than impede or block any move away from the status quo. Effective leadership in midwifery applies just as much to engendering and encouraging research as to other aspects of management. This involves recognising and supporting promising talent, giving priority to resources for research education and publicising the grants and scholarships available to midwives to fund research.

Questioning the relevance and justification for policies that have been adhered to religiously and introducing new approaches can upset the stability of an organisation, and managers may feel out of control when accepted standards are challenged. As has been pointed out earlier, however, constant evaluation and enquiry into midwifery practice are necessary to demonstrate a clearer picture of the midwife's professional role. Schurr and Turner (1982) have pointed out that:

> 'professional maturity depends on an understanding of the relationship between responsibility and personal freedom. The correct balance has to be acquired. To this must be added the capacity for independent thought. To be able to weigh up a situation and make a wise and conscientious decision is part of being responsible, but this also includes being prepared to accept the consequences for the action that follows. This is the true meaning of accountability.'

Managers need courage and fortitude in supporting independent thought and, in fact, can only claim to be leaders when people are following them.

This chapter opened by questioning whether or not research into normal childbirth had gained acceptance by professionals within the service. The evidence of growing interest in research and the results of projects undertaken by an increasing number of midwives indicate that the scene is changing. There is still a long way to go, however, in developing a firm basis of evidence to substantiate sound practices and appropriate models of care. Unless we can achieve that, the claim that no pregnancy is normal except in retrospect, which portrays the medical model of maternity care, means, in the words of Baroness Cox (1981), 'that as a practitioner in her own right, the midwife is inevitably in danger of being defined out of existence'.

REFERENCES

Ball, J. (1985) Challenging practices in midwifery. *Nursing Mirror*, **160** (29): 44–45.

Bond, S. (1981) Research – a positive contribution to practice. *Nursing Mirror*, **153** (22): 40–43.

Boyd, C. and Sellars, L. (1982) *The British Way of Birth*. London: Pan/Spastics Society.

Cartwright, A. (1979) *The Dignity of Labour: A Study of Childbirth and Induction*. London: Tavistock.

Cox, C. (1981) Bring back the midwife. *Nursing Mirror*, **153** (23): 28–30.

Department of Health and Social Security (1968) *Annual Report of the Chief Medical Officer*, Chapter 5. London: HMSO.

Department of Health and Social Security (1983) *National Health Service Management Enquiry* (Chairman: Griffiths). London: DHSS.

Hofer, M.A. (1975) *Parent–Infant Interaction*. Amsterdam: Ciba Foundation Symposium.

House of Commons (1980) *Second Report of the Social Services Committee on Perinatal and Neonatal Mortality* (Chairman: Short). London: HMSO.

Houston, M. and Weatherston, L. (1986) Creating change in midwifery: integrating theory and practice through practice-based research groups. *Midwifery*, **2**: 65–70.

Klaus, M.H. and Kennell, J.H. (1976) *Maternal–Infant Bonding*. St Louis, Missouri: C V Mosby.

Maternity Services Advisory Committee (1982) *Antenatal Care*. London: HMSO.

Maternity Services Advisory Committee (1984) *Care During Childbirth*. London: HMSO.

Maternity Services Advisory Committee (1985) *Care of the Mother and Baby*. London: HMSO.

Methven, R.C. (1982) *An Examination of the Content and Process of the Antenatal Booking Interview*. Unpublished MSc thesis, University of Manchester.

Moore, J. and Levy, V. (1981) The management of controlled cord traction related to postpartum haemorrhage. *Proceedings of Research and the Midwife Conference*, pp. 51–64. Nursing Education Research Unit, Chelsea College, University of London.

Ottoway (1979) *Change Agents at Work*. London: Associated Business Press.

Robinson, S., Golden, J. and Bradley, S. (1983) *A Study of the Role and Responsibilities of the Midwife*. Nursing Education Research Unit Report No. 1. Chelsea College, University of London.

Romney, M. (1980) Predelivery shaving: an unjustified assault? *Journal of Obstetrics and Gynaecology*, 1(1): 33–35.

Romney, M. and Gordon, H. (1981) Is your enema really necessary? *British Medical Journal*, **282**: 1269–1271.

Schurr, M.C. and Turner, J. (1982) *Nursing – Image or Reality?* London: Hodder and Stoughton.

United Kingdon Central Council for Nursing, Midwifery and Health Visiting (1986) *A Midwife's Code of Practice for Midwives Practising in the UK*. London: UKCC.

Walker, J.F. (1977) Improving maternity care by midwifery research. *Nursing Times*, **73**(38): 1489–1490.

INDEX

113